ROYAL HISTORICAL SOCIETY
STUDIES IN HISTORY
New Series

APHRODISIACS, FERTILITY AND MEDICINE IN EARLY MODERN ENGLAND

Studies in History New Series
Editorial Board

Professor Vanessa Harding (*Convenor*)
Dr D'Maris Coffman
Professor Peter Coss (*Past and Present Society*)
Professor B. Doyle (*Economic History Society*)
Dr Rachel Hammersley
Professor M. Hughes (*Honorary Treasurer*)
Professor Daniel Power
Professor Guy Rowlands
Professor Alec Ryrie
Professor Andrew Spicer (*Literary Director*)
Professor Richard Toye (*Literary Director*)

This series is supported by annual subventions from the
Economic History Society and from the Past and Present Society

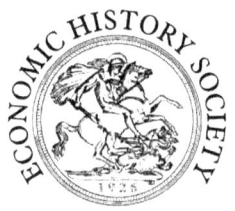

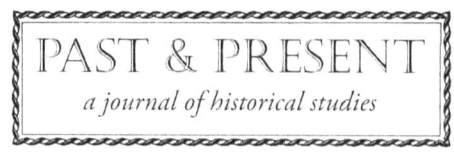

APHRODISIACS, FERTILITY AND MEDICINE IN EARLY MODERN ENGLAND

Jennifer Evans

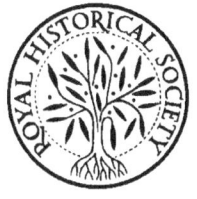

THE ROYAL HISTORICAL SOCIETY
THE BOYDELL PRESS

© Jennifer Evans 2014

All Rights Reserved. Except as permitted under current legislation no part of this work may be photocopied, stored in a retrieval system, published, performed in public, adapted, broadcast, transmitted, recorded or reproduced in any form or by any means, without the prior permission of the copyright owner

The right of Jennifer Evans to be identified as the author of this work has been asserted in accordance with sections 77 and 78 of the Copyright, Designs and Patents Act 1988

First published 2014
Paperback edition 2019

A Royal Historical Society publication
Published by The Boydell Press
an imprint of Boydell & Brewer Ltd
PO Box 9, Woodbridge, Suffolk IP12 3DF, UK
and of Boydell & Brewer Inc.
668 Mt Hope Avenue, Rochester, NY 14620–2731, USA
website: www.boydellandbrewer.com

ISBN 978–0–86193–324–2 hardback
ISBN 978–0–86193–350–1 paperback

ISSN 0269–2244

A CIP catalogue record for this book is available from the British Library

The publisher has no responsibility for the continued existence or accuracy of URLs for external or third-party internet websites referred to in this book, and does not guarantee that any content on such websites is, or will remain, accurate or appropriate

Contents

List of illustrations	vi
Acknowledgements	vii
Abbreviations	viii
Note on the text	viii
Glossary	ix
Introduction	1
1 Texts, readers and markets	29
2 The reproductive and the infertile body	51
3 Provoking lust and promoting conception	87
4 Enchanted privities and provokers of lust	131
5 Aphrodisiacs, miscarriage and menstruation	160
Conclusion	191
Bibliography	197
Index	213

Illustrations

Cover illustration: Joachim Beuckelaer, 'Market scene' (1563)
[This depicts a man propositioning a young girl set amongst a scene of indulgence in erotic foods and aphrodisiacs including cockerels, game birds and eggs.]

1. Illustration of a womb and vagina from Helkiah Crooke, *Somatographia anthropine*, London 1616 — 54
2. Illustration of a woman masturbating in a kitchen from Samuel Cock, *A voyage to Lethe*, London 1741, unpaginated — 122
3. Illustration of Marish dog stones from John Gerard, *The herball or generall historie of plantes*, London 1633 — 124

The author and publisher acknowledge with thanks the following for permission to reproduce material from their collections: the Residenzgalerie Salzburg for the cover illustration; the Wellcome Library for figure 1; the British Library for figure 2; and Archbishop Marsh's Library, Dublin, for figure 3.

Acknowledgements

I would like to offer my heartfelt gratitude to Sarah Toulalan and Alexandra Walsham for the inspiration, support, encouragement and guidance that they have given me over many years. In particular I would like to thank them for all the help and advice that they gave me on developing this research from its initial conception to completed monograph. This book would not have been possible without them or the comments and suggestions of Catherine Rider, Laura Gowing and Amanda Capern. I am also grateful to all of my colleagues and friends who have discussed, and critiqued my work including Henry French, Victoria Sparey and Victoria Bates. For guiding me through the process of publication and for patiently reading and commenting on the manuscript I am immensely grateful to Alec Ryrie and Christine Linehan.

The research for this book was funded by the University of Exeter's History Department and the Society for Renaissance Studies; without their generosity it would not have reached completion. I would also like to thank the Centre for Medical History at the University of Exeter, particularly Claire Keyte, for the intellectual and financial support that it provided for this monograph.

Parts of this book have been published in *Women's History Review* and *Social History of Medicine*, and are kindly reproduced here courtesy of Taylor & Francis and Oxford Journals. I am grateful to the reviewers commissioned for these articles whose comments strengthened and clarified some of my key arguments.

Finally I would like to thank my mum and dad, Chris and Max, for their endless love and encouragement. Their support kept me going through the good times and the stressful times and I am so grateful.

Jennifer Evans
December 2013

Abbreviations

BL   British Library, London
ODNB *Oxford Dictionary of National Biography*
OED   Oxford English Dictionary Online (www.oed.com)
WL   Wellcome Library, London

JFH   *Journal of Family History*
JHI   *Journal of the History of Ideas*
JSH   *Journal of Social History*
LPS   *Local Population Studies*
P&P   *Past & Present*
RQ   *Renaissance Quarterly*
SHM *Social History of Medicine*

Note on the Text

All quotations from contemporary printed and manuscript works retain original spellings. However, the use of 'i' and 'j', and 'u' and 'v' has been modernised. Abbreviations within the text have been expanded within square brackets. Long titles have been shortened.

Glossary

Abortifacient	A drug or other substance that induces an abortion or miscarriage.
Clyster/ Glyster	Medicines injected into the body through an orifice.
Cod	Scrotum.
Condited	To have been preserved with sugar, salt, spices, or the like. Pickled.
Confection	A substance mixed of various ingredients, or substances prepared with sugar or syrup.
Conserve	A medicinal or confectionary preparation of a plant's flowers, leaves, stalks or roots preserved with sugar.
Decoction/Apozem	A liquid in which an animal or vegetable substance has been boiled to extract the medicinal agent.
Emmenagogue	A substance that stimulates menstrual flow, and which has the power to increase or renew menstruation.
Fomentation	Flannels or cloths soaked in hot water, and often herbs, applied to the skin.
Julep	A sweet medicated drink.
Matrix	The womb.
Parturition	The act of giving birth.
Quickening	The moment at which a foetus could be felt moving inside the womb, usually around four months into pregnancy.
Recipe	A formula for the composition of a medicine or a culinary dish.
Seethed	Boiled.
Steep	To soak in water or another liquid, often milk during this period, to soften, cleanse or extract the virtues of a substance.
Suffumigation	The process of fumigating from below usually with fumes or vapours generated by burning herbs or incense.
Tansey/Tanzey	A pudding or omelette made with the juice of the tansy, a plant with a strong aromatic scent and bitter taste.
Tincture	A solution, usually in alcohol, of a principle used in medicine, chiefly vegetable but sometimes animal.

Venery	The practice or pursuit of sexual pleasure; indulgence in sexual desire.
Yard	Penis.

Introduction

Miss Bland, *Wardour Street, Soho.*
'This is a gay volatile girl; very genteel in her person; and has an extraordinary titillation in all her members; which she is very fond of increasing, by making use of provocatives for that purpose such as pullets, pigs, veal, new-laid eggs, oysters, crabs, prawns, eringoes, electuaries, &c. &c. – She is reported to have a kind of savage joy in her embraces, and sometimes leaves the marks of her penetrating teeth on her paramour's cheeks.'
Harris's list of Covent Garden ladies (1764)[1]

'Wallington "made a covenant with my eyes that I would not look upon a maid." However, his imagination and appetite were a greater threat, and these he attempted to tame by collecting scriptural passages that condemned "adultery, fornication, uncleanness, wantonness" and the seductions of "strong women," by working hard at his calling, by fasting and arising "betimes in the morning," and by "abstaining from divers meats as eggs and oysters and wine and many other things which I loved very well".'
Paul Seaver, *Wallington's world* (1985)[2]

'When he came home She gave him Kisses,
and Sack-Posset very good:
Caudles too, she never misses,
for they warm, and heat the Blood.
Such things will Create desire,
and new kindle *Cupid's* fire,
These things made him kiss his Wife,
And to call her Love and Life.' *The London cuckold* (1685–8)[3]

These diverse quotations exemplify the many surprising and socially complex ways in which aphrodisiacs were understood in early modern England. *Harris's list of Covent Garden ladies*, written by Samuel Derrick, claimed to describe actual women working as prostitutes in London in the eighteenth century. This particular listing for a 'volatile girl' immediately emphasises the great many foods that were described as sexually stimulating, and notes their connection to pleasurable sexual encounters. The substances, in this instance and in many others, were listed by the author without any expla-

---

[1] Hallie Rubenhold (ed.), *The harlot's handbook, Harris's list*, Stroud 2007, 155–6.
[2] Paul S. Seaver, *Wallington's world: a Puritan artisan in seventeenth-century London*, Stanford 1985, 26–7.
[3] Anon., *The London cuckold*, London 1685–8.

nation, suggesting that the, predominantly male, audience was expected to know these foods by reputation and comprehend the effects that they would have upon the body. The ubiquitous understanding of the humoural medical system provided the most accessible means for interpreting the actions of these foods and, as this book will demonstrate, was the main way in which aphrodisiacs were categorised across the early modern era. Finally this advertisement implies that, as well as understanding the role of these substances in the promotion of sexual behaviour, men of a certain wealth may have been willing to pay for a sexual encounter that incorporated the stimulating properties that these foods were thought to provide.

Similarly the extract from the diary of the Puritan artisan Nehemiah Wallington (1598–1658) demonstrates that many aphrodisiacs were a common element of the everyday diet. As this book will go on to establish, many of the simples and compounds thought to increase lust and to enhance the generative body (the body as it relates to generation/reproduction) were ingredients common to herb gardens and hedgerows and in some cases were staples of the early modern diet. As an ordinary part of the early modern regimen, it could be argued that these substances were only understood to serve as sexual stimulants in particular contexts, such as the encounter with a prostitute described above. Yet Wallington's desire to remove them from his diet reflects a belief in their stimulating properties as inherent to the way in which they worked upon the body, regardless of specific need. Moreover, his inclusion of this group of foods with his other measures of restraint demonstrates the intimate relationship that existed between the consumption of foods, the constitution of the body, and one's moral and social character.

Finally, the extract from the ballad *The London cuckold* highlights that aphrodisiacs were most commonly understood within the framework of marriage and procreation. In this ballad the sexually unsatisfied wife, who is yet to be made a mother, feeds stimulating foods to her husband to try to encourage him to fulfil his marital duties. Although it is not made explicit here, part of this marital role was to produce offspring who would confirm the place of the husband and wife in their social roles. Aphrodisiacs were at this time almost ubiquitously understood as medicaments for infertility. Moreover, that ballads such as this one discussed and described aphrodisiacs demonstrates that they were widely understood in early modern society; ballads had to be accessible and reference ideas with which a wide cross-section of society would identify. Thus, from these extracts it is apparent that early modern men and women understood that a range of foods and medicines could be sexually stimulating and that they could potentially be used in a range of circumstances to regulate sexual desire, behaviour and fertility.

This book will chart the various ways in which aphrodisiacs were understood in this period and in particular how they were thought to affect the reproductive organs. It will be argued that aphrodisiacs were regarded as a treatment for barrenness and impotence across the sixteenth, seventeenth and eighteenth centuries. That they were believed to work in this way accentuates the inextricable link between procreation and sexual pleasure that existed in early modern medical theory. Although this book will focus primarily on the theoretical discussion of the virtues of aphrodisiacs it will also show that, at least sometimes, men and women in early modern England used these substances in the ways described in medical and popular literature both to enhance their sexual experiences and also to improve their chances of conceiving. The familiarity and availability of some of these herbs, spices and foods makes this all the more likely. However, with the limited evidence presented in surviving early modern documents it is not possible to make any certain claims about the scale of the actual use of these substances.

'Provokers of lust', 'Provokers of venery' and 'Aphrodisiacks'

Throughout this book sexual stimulants are referred to by a variety of terms which reflect the language use of early modern medical writers. Additionally for ease of reading they are described as aphrodisiacs. For much of the period medical and botanical writers defined stimulating substances as provokers of lust or provokers of venery: venery meaning the practice or pursuit of sexual pleasure and the indulgence of sexual desire.[4] These terms – 'venereal' and 'venery' – originated from the Latin and related to the Roman goddess of beauty and sensual love, Venus. This reflected the fact that Galenic and other Greek medical works were often translated into Latin at this time. In other areas of reproductive medicine the tendency to use Latinate terms was also true: the labels used for menstrual bleeding (menstrua) and abnormal vaginal discharge (fluor albus), for example, were both Latin terms. However, in the late seventeenth and early eighteenth century scholars discussing reproduction and generation started also to include or use Greek terms: menstrua became catamena and the fluor albus became Leucorrhoea.[5] Similarly the

---

[4] OED, s.v. 'Venery', accessed 13 Aug. 2013. 'Aphrodisiac' does not seem to have been recorded in any other seventeenth-century dictionary.

[5] Sara Read, *Menstruation and the female body in early modern England*, Basingstoke 2013, 28, 195 n. 29. R. W. McConchie has noted that many words of classical origin that had been naturalised into English were in the sixteenth century re-alienated and given new neoclassical forms. He argued that there was no difference in semantic clarity between the English and classical forms. The change was often motivated by the prestige of classical learning and to allow words to be protected from the corruption of popular use. Although occurring a century later, and between Latin and Greek rather than English, this interpretation may provide some explanation for the changes seen in the late seventeenth century: *Lexicography and physic: the record of sixteenth-century English medical terminology*, Oxford 1997, 66–71. The late adoption of Greek terms may also reflect that many Greek authors of note were only slowly translated over the sixteenth and seventeenth centuries: L. D. Reynolds and N. G. Wilson, *Scribes and scholars: a guide to the transmission of Greek and Latin literature*, Oxford 1974, 148–52. Similarly there were only a handful of Greek medical texts available in printed form during the sixteenth century when modern anatomy was being developed: Vivian Nutton, "'Prisci

language for sexual stimulants in some treatises also changed, adopting words that were derived from the Greek equivalent to Venus, Aphrodite, such as aphrodisiac(k). This change was not comprehensive; Latin terms were not suddenly or gradually superseded by Greek ones, nor did it reflect a fundamental shift in how these substances were understood or believed to work. It is also not clear what provoked the sudden appearance of Greek terminology in this field.[6] The earliest appearances of 'aphrodisiac' in English language treatises can be seen in the works of Theophile Bonet (1684), a Swiss physician, John Jones (1701), a lawyer and physician in Wales, John Marten (1709), a surgeon, and Thomas Fuller (1710), an extra-licentiate of the Royal College of Physicians.[7] Even in these texts the adoption of Greek terminology was not always consistent. Jean Astruc wrote in 1743 of 'Remedia Aphrodisiaca', but throughout his treatise relied heavily on Latin terminology.[8] Yet, Astruc also clarified that these were not a new or distinct taxonomy of medicaments as he explained that they 'are met with almost in all medicinal Books'.[9] Bonet likewise suggested that there was no distinction between those things described as a provoker to venery and those described as an aphrodisiac: first, he provided a description of the characteristics of aphrodisiacs that correlates with the main categories of stimulant examined in this book – which were described throughout the period as provokers of venery.[10] Secondly, he used the word 'venery' throughout his discussion of

---

dissectionum professores"': Greek texts and renaissance anatomists', in A. C. Dionisotti, Anthony Grafton and Jill Kraye (eds), *The uses of Greek and Latin: historical essays*, London 1988, 111–26 at p. 114.

[6] I am grateful to Alexandra Walsham, Jonathan Barry and Sarah Toulalan for their thoughts on this issue.

[7] The OED erroneously dates the use of this term to 1710: OED s.v. 'Aphrodisiac', accessed 26 July 2010. See Theophile Bonet, *Mercurius compitalitius: or, A guide to the practical physician*, London [1682] 1684, 545, 694–5; John Jones, *The mysteries of opium reveal'd*, London 1701, 52; John Marten, *Gonosologium novum: or, a new system of all the secret infirmities and diseases, natural, accidental, and venereal in men and women*, London 1709, 49; and Thomas Fuller, *Pharmacopoia extemporanea: or, A body of prescripts*, London 1710, 133. The sixteenth-century dictionary of Thomas Elyot included 'Aphrodisia' as days or sacrifices to Venus or venereal pastimes, 'Aphrodisium' as an image of Venus and 'Aphrodisius' as a prelate or disciple of St Peter, but made no reference to aphrodisiac: *Bibliotheca Eliotae*, London 1559, s.v. 'Aphrodisia', 'Aphrodisium' and 'Aphrodisius'. One Greek dictionary noted that feasts dedicated to Aphrodite were called *Aphrodisiana* but did not include the term aphrodisiac: Pierre Danet, *A complete dictionary of the Greek and Roman antiquities*, London 1700, s.v. 'Aphrodite'. Aphrodite appears in several dictionaries including *The great historical, geographical and poetical dictionary*, which states that she was born of the sea and that led some to think that moisture was a crucial part of generation: Louis Moreiri, *The great historical, geographical and poetical dictionary*, London 1694, s.v. 'Aphrodite'.

[8] Jean Astruc, *A treatise on all the diseases incident to women*, London 1743, 345.

[9] Ibid.

[10] Bonet, *Mercurius compitalitius*, 694.

these substances; in particular he noted that aphrodisiacks were 'those things indeed that excite the Spirits stir up Venery'.[11]

The move towards this particular term may also have been related to the rise in printed materials discussing venereal disease. As is apparent from its name, much of the discussion of this disorder and the drugs (anti-venereals) that were used to cure it drew upon naturalised Latin terms. In one very rare example, Stephen Blankaart's seventeenth-century *Physical dictionary* included the terms *Aphrodisius morbus* and *Lues venerea* (venereal disease) as synonymous.[12] A few eighteenth-century authors also connected this disease and 'aphrodisiac'. In 1736 a version of Luigi Luisini's *Aphrodisiacus* was published in English with a preface by the surgeon and physician Daniel Turner, who had already published several treatises on venereal disease.[13] It is not apparent what 'aphrodisiacus' meant, or how it was being used: the Oxford English Dictionary does not record this as a part of the English lexicon. However, this work was a collection of all the historical writers who had written about venereal disease. The 1755 edition of Samuel Johnson's dictionary also explained that 'APRHODISIACAL' and 'APRHODISIACK' related to the venereal disease.[14] Moreover, Johnson made no reference to sexual stimulation. It may be that the surge of interest in venereal disease in the seventeenth century encouraged the introduction of this term. Nonetheless, it is not clear what reasons would have motivated this. Moreover, the understanding that aphrodisiacs were specifically a treatment for venereal disease was not as widespread as the understanding that these substances were synonymous with provokers of venery.

The term aphrodisiac was thus a new one in the early modern period, one that was only gradually being adopted in the latter part of the period. Although it will be seen that aphrodisiacs were understood in a way that is recognisable to modern audience – they stimulated sexual desire – it is also important to emphasise at the outset that the early modern mind-set was not the same as our own. In modern society it is accepted that a person's mental and emotional state can affect their physical well-being: stress, for example, is known to cause physical problems and symptoms. This was true in the early modern period as well. A person's emotional and physiological states were thought to be closely connected. The various constitutions of the humoural body were thought to predispose people to certain emotions

---

[11] Ibid.

[12] Stephen Blankaart, *A physical dictionary in which all the terms relating either to anatomy, chirurgery … are very accurately explain'd*, London 1684, 23. I have not come across this terminology for the venereal disease anywhere else.

[13] Luigi Luisini, *Aphrodisiacus: containing a summary of the ancient writers on the venereal disease*, London 1736; ODNB, s.v. 'Daniel Turner', accessed 11 Apr. 2013. This word only appears in the title of the book.

[14] Samuel Johnson, *A dictionary of the English language*, London 1755–6, s.v. 'Aphrodisiacal' and 'Aphrodisiack'.

such as anger, desire or melancholy. Moreover, it was believed that a range of illnesses could result in altered emotional states, or that altered emotional states could lead to physical illness. However, it has been claimed that in the eighteenth century a 'modern' attitude towards sexuality developed, as a part of which sexual desire and pleasure became divorced from reproduction.[15] Yet, as will be shown in this book, between 1550 and 1780 descriptions of aphrodisiacs implicitly accepted and explicitly described lust as an integral part of conception and generation. This is not to say that in other areas the two did not start to separate, but that in medical and popular understandings aphrodisiacs were never only substances that stimulated lust. They were medicines that functioned as a remedy for infertility: the ways in which they were thought to stimulate lust made the generative body more fertile and were thought to improve the chances of conceiving. Consequently lust throughout this period was seen as central to reproductive sex, and sexual pleasure could not be separated from the generative nature of sexual intercourse.

Options for treating infertility

When talking about barrenness, medical texts throughout the early modern period often cited the biblical tale of Rachel, who was unable to conceive, in order to emphasise the distressing nature of this medical problem. Jane Sharp, for example, cited Rachel's words to Jacob '*Give me Children or else I die*'.[16] Robert Johnson's treatise *The practice of physick* also included Rachel's lament alongside the observation that there were 'very few Women in a Marriage state but desire Children, yea some would give all they have in the world for a Child, and are very impatient if they do not Conceive'.[17] These descriptions offer a brief insight into the anguish, despair and longing that infertility (commonly termed barrenness or unfruitfulness in the early modern period) could cause women, and men. Infertility, as Daphna Oren-Magidor has highlighted, did not only refer to complete childlessness. Men and women who struggled to conceive, but eventually did have a child, were thought to be infertile up until the point of conception. Similarly those couples who had had children previously but subsequently struggled

---

[15] Thomas Laqueur, 'Orgasm, generation, and the politics of reproductive biology', *Representations: The Making of the Modern Body: Sexuality and Society in the Nineteenth Century* xiv (1986), 1–41 at p. 1; Faramerz Dabhoiwala, *The origins of sex: a history of the first sexual revolution*, Oxford 2012, 141–4.

[16] Jane Sharp, *The midwives book: or The whole art of midwifry discovered*, London 1671, 177.

[17] Robert Johnson, *Praxis medicinae reformata: or, The practice of physic reformed*, London 1700, 245.

to conceive were also thought to be barren or infertile.[18] Anxieties about infertility resonated with cultural and social ideals about the social roles of men and women and with notions about the institutions of marriage and the family. Men and women who found themselves unable to conceive consequently undertook a variety of therapeutic regimes to remedy the problem. This book will focus on the understanding and consumption of aphrodisiacs, because they represent a consistent, ubiquitous and common approach to the disorder. However, this is not to suggest that they were the only means of curing infertility discussed in the period, nor even that they were the most popular. As with the majority of disorders in the early modern period, Galenic medicine suggested that to remedy any form of infertility the body's humours had to be rebalanced and any underlying distemper of the womb, testicles or genitalia had to be remedied. Culpeper, for example, included therapeutic regimes for a range of uterine distempers damaging to a woman's fertility.[19] Aphrodisiacs were only one element of this therapeutic response to infertility.

In addition to the internal medicines offered for the cure of infertility, many women, including Catherine of Braganza, utilised the healing properties of baths and spas to remedy their infertility (there is no evidence of men using baths for this purpose).[20] In the *Bath memoirs* of Robert Pierce it was recorded that

> we come now to *Marry'd Women*, and we begin with those which never had a Child, till render'd fruitful by the *Bath*: And this is an Effect of *bathing*, so very well known already, and so generally assented to, that when any one comes hither that is Childless, they presently say that *She comes for the common Cause*.[21]

So potent did Pierce think the baths to be that he went on to suggest that several women had attended the baths for other ailments only to find themselves 'unexpectedly, prov'd fruitful afterwards'.[22] The baths appear to have been popular with the aristocracy, though the expense of travelling to the baths and lodgings during the treatment perhaps proved too much for those who were less well off. The baths themselves were thought to work in ways that reflected some of the aphrodisiac treatments, in particular in penetrating the reproductive organs and supplying them with heat. The author of *Dr Carr's medicinal epistles* (1714), John Quincy, did not believe that this heat

---

[18] Daphna Oren-Magidor, '"Make me a fruitfull vine": dealing with infertility in early modern England', unpubl. PhD diss. Brown 2012, introduction.

[19] Nicholas Culpeper, *Culpeper's directory for midwives: or, A guide for women*, London 1662.

[20] Oren-Magidor, '"Fruitfull vine"', ch. v.

[21] Robert Pierce, *Bath memoirs: or, Observations in three and forty years practice, at the bath, what cures have been there wrought*, Bristol 1697, 195.

[22] Ibid. 196.

stimulated sexual desire, but did argue that it was very conducive to opening obstructions that prevented conception.[23]

As this book will argue, medical writers advocated aphrodisiacs as a remedy for infertility because it was widely acknowledged that a loss of sexual desire inhibited conception. Yet medical practitioners also offered further advice on how to encourage sexual activity and stimulate lost libido. Philip Barrough suggested that men who suffered a loss of sex drive should sleep in a soft bed and should 'reade things that doe stirre up thinges carnal'.[24] Similarly the sixteenth-century surgeon Ambrose Paré declared that women could be stimulated by their husbands in a variety of ways:

> When the husband commeth into his wives chamber hee must entertaine her with all kinde of dalliance, wanton behaviour, and allurements to venery: but if he perceive her to be slow, and more cold, he must cherish, embrace, and tickle her, and shall not abruptly, the nerves being suddenly distended, breake into the field of nature, but rather shall creepe in by little and little, intermixing more wanton kisses with wanton words and speeches, handling her secret parts and dugs, that she may take fire and bee enflamed to venery.[25]

At the end of this discussion Paré included the use of aphrodisiacs for those women who were particularly disinclined to engage in intercourse.

Clearly aphrodisiacs were not the only means by which men and women could seek to improve their fertility. For those who suffered from an identifiable disease which happened to result in barrenness, such as the whites (an excessive flow of vaginal discharge that was frequently described as resulting in barrenness), treatment would most likely have followed the precepts designed to remove that particular distemper. Nonetheless, it is also clear that aphrodisiacs were an important part of the way in which early modern men and women conceptualised the treatment of infertility. They represent an important element of the sexual and reproductive health discourse of early modern England, one that to this point has been relatively neglected or glossed over as trivial or titillating.

Aphrodisiacs in history

Although scholars have touched upon the subject of aphrodisiacs in early modern England, this has tended to be in the form of passing references to the use of particular substances, often with reference to certain people

---

[23] John Quincy, *Dr. Carr's medicinal epistles*, London 1714, 55.
[24] Philip Barrough, *The methode of phisicke, conteyning the causes, signes, and cures of inward diseases in mans bodie from the head to the foote*, London 1583, 142.
[25] Ambrose Paré, *The works of that famous chirurgion Ambrose Parey*, London 1634, 889.

or the courts of certain monarchs.[26] There has been little analysis of these substances in detail or consideration of their wider role in reproduction. More commonly discussions of the early modern period have been included in works that consider a range of historical periods, which has limited the investigation of the peculiarities of early modern stimulants to a single chapter. Nevertheless, these works have drawn attention to the interest of past cultures in provoking lust and have raised interesting questions about their role in medicine and society.

Several early works that considered aphrodisiacs approached the topic from an antiquarian point of view. In 1930 Henri Stearns Denninger published 'A history of substances known as aphrodisiacs',[27] a brief article which traced the history of provocatives from the Egyptians, Greeks and Romans through to the Middle Ages and then the nineteenth and twentieth centuries. Alan Hull Walton took a similar approach in his 1958 book *Aphrodisiacs: from legend to prescription* which also traced the history of these substances across several temporal boundaries. These works predominantly focused on the development of aphrodisiacs from their earliest roots in ancient societies. Furthermore, works such as these and Hull Walton's 1965 edition of John Davenport's *Aphrodisiacs* (1869) were written salaciously for a diverse contemporary audience.[28] They not only listed many substances that were previously considered to be aphrodisiacs but ones which could potentially still be employed. These authors did not seek to understand the medical functions of the substances that they discussed, but described aphrodisiacs only in terms of lust and desire as their intended audience expected. Denninger provided his readers with a concise, almost list-like, account of many substances considered to be aphrodisiacs in the Middle Ages and the Renaissance.[29] However, at no point did he explain why these foods were considered to be stimulating. Instead, he only wrote that 'During the Renaissance the public was, to say the least, rather voluptuous, and aphrodisiacs were equally common in the household and in the apothecary shops.'[30] Walton also noted the variety and commonality of aphrodisiacs. Both of these authors represented the early modern period as being particularly lascivious

---

[26] Ivan Bloch, *Sexual life in England past and present*, London 1958, 301–7; Thomas Laqueur, *Making sex: body and gender from the Greeks to Freud*, Cambridge MA–London 1990, 102–3; Michael J. O'Dowd, *The history of medications for women: materia medica woman*, New York–London 2001, 23, 38, 58, 114, 160.

[27] Henri Stearns Denninger, 'A history of substances known as aphrodisiacs', *Annales of Medical History* ii/4 (1930), 383–93.

[28] John Davenport, *Aphrodisiacs and love stimulants with other chapters on the secrets of Venus*, ed. with intro. and notes Alan Hull Walton, London 1965.

[29] Stearns Denninger, 'A history of substances known as aphrodisiacs', 388. He includes discussions of eryngo, mandrake root, zedoary, ginger, pepper, cumin, clove, vanilla and sparrow's brains.

[30] Ibid. 389.

and aphrodisiacal. Nonetheless, Walton did attempt to understand the ways in which early modern substances worked. Unfortunately, his interpretation was based on the anachronistic imposition of contemporary categories on the foods that he was discussing. He explained that there were two main types of substance which would provoke sexual desire: ones which excited the senses and produced a physical capability or desire, and those which clouded the wits and banished self-control.[31] Such categories do not correlate with early modern descriptions of aphrodisiacs, even though many of the substances that medical writers described could be thought of in this way. The analysis presented in this book is only interested in the ways in which early modern men and women understood these substances, not in whether they would actually have worked or not. Although it may be possible to assess the effects some of these substances have on the body, as John Riddle has attempted to do for ancient contraceptives and abortifacients, this approach is problematic. First, it assumes that early modern reproductive bodies were the same as our own, which the differing nutritional standards of early modern diets would suggest is not always true. Moreover, even if modern science can identify the effects of some plants, we cannot always know whether they were consumed in quantities that would have meant that these effects were felt. Finally, we cannot always assume to know how in the past these substances were prepared, and consequently know whether this affected the efficacy of particular plants.[32] What matters therefore, is how these plants were perceived, described and recorded, as this tells us what people believed was effective, how these understandings tied in with their broader social and cultural beliefs and how they responded to particular medical issues.

The focus of these authors on excess is perhaps one of the ways in which they sought to titillate their readers. In some cases it seems that Davenport's interest was restricted to examples where consumption of a substance such as cantharides, chocolate and opium had such excessive and damaging effects.[33] Similarly the assertion that aphrodisiacs, particularly those influenced by ancient medicine, were relatively consistent across cultures and historical periods, suggests a form of common sexual understanding between all historic cultures and societies, which reflects both the salacious and antiquarian themes of these works. Although it will be argued here that aphrodisiacs were commonly understood and widely discussed, it is not being claimed, as these works do, that these substances were only consumed to

---

[31] Alan Hull Walton, *Aphrodisiacs from legend to prescription: a study of aphrodisiacs throughout the ages, with sections on suitable food, glandular extracts, hormone stimulation and rejuvenation*, Westport, CN 1958, 97.

[32] John Riddle, *Contraception and abortion from the ancient world to the Renaissance*, Cambridge, MA–London 1992, 32–6, and *Eve's herbs: a history of contraception and abortion in the West*, Cambridge MA–London 1997, 47–50. Further problems arise from the fact that the tests that Riddle cites were mostly conducted on rats.

[33] Davenport, *Aphrodisiacs and love stimulants*, 35, 40, 46.

excite excessive sexual appetites. Rather, that for many early modern men and women, using these substances to provoke sexual desire was considered to be a way of improving fertility.

Aphrodisiacs have also been discussed indirectly in broader studies such as Philippa Pullar's *Consuming passions* (1970). Pullar examined English foods and appetites and only included a brief discussion of aphrodisiacs as an appendix to the work.[34] However, although she started this description by imposing modern understandings of desire upon the past, she did note the inherent connection between fertility and sexual potency.[35] Nonetheless, when considering the past Pullar argued that ideas about erotic foods were based only on the doctrine of signatures and the foods 'newness' or exoticism.[36] Broader studies of the history of generation and the family have also touched upon the place of aphrodisiacs in early modern society. In *Obstetrics and gynaecology in Tudor and Stuart England* (1982) Audrey Eccles discussed 'sexuality and conception', although she only recorded the use of windy foods to help male sexual incapacity.[37] Similarly Helen Berry and Elizabeth Foyster have examined the subject of infertility, particularly male, and have highlighted that there was a range of medicines designed to increase lust, and help conception.[38] Berry and Foyster, however, suggested that men's sexual techniques, rather than aphrodisiacs, were portrayed as central to their ability to give women pleasure, and so maximise their chances of having children.[39] Without disputing their argument, this book will also show that many aphrodisiacs were thought to be able to help men maintain tumescence and prevent premature ejaculation. These substances could also increase female pleasure substantially by invigorating the male seed with heat and vital spirits which titillated the female generative system upon contact. Thus aphrodisiacs were believed to help improve certain aspects of male sexual performance in order to enhance the chances of conception.

Perhaps the most important works that have addressed the topic of aphrodisiacs are those of Angus McLaren. He devoted a chapter in *Reproductive rituals* (1984) to the remedy of barrenness and the promotion of generation, outlining the link between procreation and pleasure and a basic frame-

---

[34] Philippa Pullar, *Consuming passions: a history of English food and appetites*, London 1970, 235–40.
[35] Ibid. 235.
[36] Ibid. 237.
[37] Audrey Eccles, *Obstetrics and gynaecology in Tudor and Stuart England*, London–Canberra 1982, 33–42 at p. 36.
[38] Helen Berry and Elizabeth Foyster, 'Childless men in early modern England', in Helen Berry and Elizabeth Foyster (eds), *The family in early modern England*, Cambridge 2007, 158–83 at p. 172.
[39] Ibid. 172.

work for the ways in which aphrodisiacs were understood.[40] Yet McLaren claimed that provoking lust was a mainly male concern and that remedies for female barrenness warmed and invigorated, but did not necessary stir lust.[41] Although his work provides an invaluable introduction to this topic, much of his evidence was drawn from literary sources and so obscures the detailed medical understanding of these substances. Nonetheless, McLaren did show that understandings of sexual stimulation were widespread and existed beyond the realm of printed medical treatises. McLaren discussed aphrodisiacs as just one element of sexual practice alongside the timing of intercourse and issues to do with pregnancy. This situates aphrodisiacs well within the broader framework of obstetrics and gynaecology but did not allow for a detailed investigation of the peculiarities of these substances. In his 2007 work *Impotence* McLaren again utilised a range of sources to examine the ways in which 'fumbling' men in early modern England were mocked and ridiculed.[42] Again, although McLaren described the herbal aphrodisiacs recommended by Nicholas Culpeper, aphrodisiacs did not form the central theme of his analysis.[43] McLaren's broad discussions did not provide specific details about the way in which the understandings of aphrodisiacs shifted and changed across the period, neither did he consider the sexed and gendered nature of these substances, although *Impotence* did consider the ways in which specifically male sexual failure was ridiculed and portrayed in early modern culture. Here I will consider how changing ideas about the sexed body interacted with the understanding of aphrodisiacs, and how aphrodisiacs were evaluated across the period in light of new anatomical understandings of the body.

In contrast to McLaren's broad approach, Valeria Finucci's 2008 article 'There's the rub: searching for sexual remedies in the New World' specifically addressed the search for a sexual stimulant by Duke Vincenzo Gonzaga of Mantua's apothecary.[44] Finucci recorded numerous kinds of aphrodisiacs available in early modern Europe including those that operated through the doctrine of signatures, talismans and exotic foods.[45] Finucci did explain the medicinal value of some of these substances; however, most of the article merely recites the many things that could be purchased. Such case studies are valuable chiefly for revealing the interest with which certain early modern men and women could view aphrodisiacs, and for highlighting their relevance as a subject of enquiry.

---

[40] Angus McLaren, *Reproductive rituals: the perception of fertility in England from the sixteenth century to the nineteenth century*, London–New York 1984, 31.
[41] Ibid. 38.
[42] Idem, *Impotence: a cultural history*, Chicago–London 2007, ch. iii.
[43] Ibid. 57, 80.
[44] Valeria Finucci, '"There's the rub": searching for sexual remedies in the new world', *Journal of Medieval and Early Modern Studies* xxxviii/3 (2008), 523–57.
[45] Ibid. 529–31.

INTRODUCTION

This book provides a middle ground to previous studies, considering the peculiarities of sexual stimulants in the context of one country and in one time period. Many of the studies discussed repeated that certain substances at one time or another functioned to promote lust. But in this way aphrodisiacs become dehistoricised by the suggestion that at all times they function in the same way: lust and its stimulation is understood as a universal constant that prioritises the emotional over the bodily and reproductive. Moreover, it obscures the culturally specific understandings of these substances, in this case as fertility treatments. In the early modern period the stimulation of lust, as it was understood through the humoural model, prioritised the connection between pleasure and procreation. Aphrodisiacs were always, then, more than curiosities or consumables but were instead an integral part of early modern sexual health practices.

Historical contexts

Beyond this rather narrow field of study, this book also draws upon and contributes to two broader contextual frameworks. Firstly, the demographic discussions of fertility rates across the period and, secondly, the religious and familial context of infertility, including masculinity and sexuality.

Demographic fertility trends

Several historians have investigated the shifting fertility trends of early modern England. Tim Hitchcock, drawing on the work of Tony Wrigley and Roger Schofield, summarised that the period between 1650 and 1750 was characterised by stagnant population growth caused by late marriage and reduced fertility.[46] This started to change around 1701 when the age of marriage began to fall, yet a subsequent increase in fertility did not become apparent until after 1750.[47] As Helen Berry and Elizabeth Foyster have suggested, demographic and economic trends, whether explicitly understood or not, were likely to have framed social attitudes towards reproduction.[48] Hence the low fertility rate of the period was reflected in the interest shown by medical writers, and the broader populace, in the causes of, and cures for, infertility. The almost ubiquitous discussion of barrenness, impotence and aphrodisiacs found in early modern medical texts demonstrates that English society recognised the difficulties associated with successful conception and were concerned with remedies and dietary regimens that would enhance chances of producing progeny.

One of the main reasons why population levels began to increase in the latter part of the period was the lowering of the age of marriage – marrying

---

[46] Tim Hitchcock, *English sexualities, 1700–1800*, Basingstoke–London 1997, 25.
[47] Ibid. 26.
[48] Berry and Foyster, 'Childless men', 163.

at an earlier age meant that people spent a greater part of their childbearing years in a sexual relationship that could legitimately result in children.[49] Pier Paolo Viazzo has also suggested that overall population levels changed because of a reduction in mortality rates and a marked rise in the birth rate.[50] The upswing in fertility measured across the early modern period was a key consideration in the periodisation of my research; it would perhaps be presumed that as the period progressed people may have become aware that more people were having children. If these changes in fertility and population levels were noticed by those at the time it might be expected that the need to discuss infertility, infertility treatments and aphrodisiacs would have lessened in the latter part of the period. It is evident for example that eighteenth-century herbals included fewer aphrodisiacs than their earlier counterparts. However, medical treatises continued to discuss infertility at length. This was likely in part because a rise in fertility overall was scant consolation or comfort for those who did find themselves childless and struggling to conceive; it may even have made their own situation seem more exceptional and thus more distressing. The continued frequency with which infertility was discussed and the length at which it was described and remedies for it advocated, also suggests that throughout the eighteenth century medical writers perceived this to be a topic of widespread concern.

Alternatively, Wrigley has suggested that the increased fertility rates later in the period could be attributed to a reduction in the number of pregnancies that resulted in stillbirth.[51] It is important then to recognise that the moment of conception was only one part of the reproductive process. Gestation and parturition also had to be successfully negotiated in order for a living child to be born. Early modern society believed that pregnancy was a precarious condition; miscarriage could be induced by a variety of different causes. The final chapter of this book therefore considers whether aphrodisiacs were ever thought to play a role in strengthening the body beyond the moment of conception. It is evident, however, that although conception and miscarriage were considered to be two closely connected facets of fertility, aphrodisiacs were not often advocated to help maintain a pregnancy.

Demographers like Richard T. Vann have also cautioned scholars to consider the possibility that fertility rates in particular locations were artificially reduced by human action, the use of contraceptive practices known as

[49] Tim Hitchcock, 'The reformulation of sexual knowledge in eighteenth-century England', *Signs* xxxvii/4 (2012) 823–32 at p. 823.

[50] Pier Paolo Viazzo, 'Mortality, fertility, and family', trans. Caroline Beamish, in David I. Kertzer and Marzio Barbagli (eds), *The history of the European family*, I: *Family life in early modern times, 1500–1789*, New Haven–London 2001, 157–87 at p. 163.

[51] E. A. Wrigley, 'Explaining the rise in marital fertility in England in the "long" eighteenth century', *Economic History Review* li/3 (1998), 435–64 at pp. 452–3. Wrigley argued (p. 440) that this was connected to maternal nutrition and changes in delivery skills and childbed practices.

family limitation strategies. Vann has argued that the demographic data for Colyton in Devon suggests that before 1750 families were using prolonged lactation in order to reduce the number of children that they conceived.[52] Dorothy McLaren has also demonstrated that wet-nurses in Chesham had fewer children across their married life than wealthy women who put their children out to nurse, and that there was an awareness that '"prolonged suckling hindereth propogation"'.[53] While it is important to establish the use of contraceptive strategies by early modern men and women, assuming that all of the instances where families had a substantial gap between births, or a lower number of births than expected, was as a result of deliberate intervention is perhaps misguided. The focus of demographic scholars and scholars of reproduction on birth control is perhaps anachronistic and influenced by modern preoccupations. Importantly it obscures the strongly pro-natalist attitude of early modern England.[54] The concern with which medical writers discussed infertility, both absolute and temporary, and the ways in which the wider populace also expressed concern about the difficulties of conceiving paints a very different picture, where couples genuinely struggled to conceive, even if they had previously had children. The qualitative evidence would thus suggest that in many cases men and women's fertility was dictated by poor reproductive health as much as it was by deliberate strategies of family limitation.

Concerns about fertility were likely not only driven by anxieties about conceiving, but about the number of children that survived to adulthood. Demographers have shown that levels of child and infant mortality were relatively high during the sixteenth and seventeenth centuries (around 200 deaths per 1,000 births).[55] High levels of child mortality have been identified in York, Wrangle (Lincolnshire) and Broughton (Lancashire).[56] Conversely Peter Razzell and Christine Spence have argued that child mortality rates were relatively low in London between 1550 and 1650, although they still noted that the overall rate between the middle of the sixteenth and middle

---

[52] Richard. T. Vann 'Unnatural infertility, or, whatever happened in Colyton? Some reflections on *English population history from family reconstitution, 1580–1837*', *Continuity and Change* xiv/1 (1999), 91–104 at pp. 95, 100–1.

[53] Dorothy McLaren, 'Nature's contraceptive: wet-nursing and prolonged lactation: the cases of Chesham, Buckinghamshire, 1578–1601, *Medical History* xxiii/4 (1979), 426–41 at pp. 433–4.

[54] Oren-Magidor, '"Fruitfull vine"', introduction.

[55] R. E. Jones, 'Further evidence on the decline in infant mortality in pre-industrial England: North Shropshire, 1561–1810', *Population Studies* xxxiv/2 (1980), 239–50 at at pp. 239–40.

[56] See Chris Galley, 'A never-ending succession of epidemics? Mortality in early-modern York', *SHM* vii/1 (1994), 29–57; Andy Gritt, 'Mortality crisis and household structure: an analysis of parish registers and Compton census, Broughton, Lancashire, 1667–1676', *LPS* lxxix (2007), 38–65; Dorothy McLaren, 'Fertility, infant mortality, and breastfeeding in the seventeenth century', *Medical History* xxii/4 (1978), 378–96.

of the eighteenth century more than doubled.[57] Numerous diseases have been identified as responsible for the deaths of so many children. In addition to outbreaks of plague, it has been argued that urban areas were susceptible to infectious diseases and epidemic infantile diarrhoea.[58] Moreover, variations in mortality rates have suggested that numerous children died from respiratory diseases in the winter and intestinal diseases in the summer.[59] Diseases such as smallpox and measles were also likely to kill many children.[60] All of these perils meant that, as Chris Galley has noted for York, 'roughly one in four infants died during their first year of life and barely one in two survived to reach fifteen' years old.[61] It is probable therefore that many men and women would have been aware of the potential for children to contract disease, and subsequently die early in life. Even though these trends may not have been fully understood at the time, early modern society acknowledged that children frequently died, and often died very young, encouraging men and women, particularly of the higher classes, to hope for multiple children. In this situation, concerns about fertility and the ability to conceive would again have applied both to those suffering from absolute infertility and those who had children but were struggling to conceive again.

Galley also explained in his study of York that the stillbirth rate during the early modern period was relatively high and additionally that many of the deaths recorded can be classified as endogenous (not caused by external factors such as disease) occurring early in life.[62] This again was reflected in the attitude of early modern medical writers to conception and fertility. William Salmon, for example, argued that 'such as are Barren, either bear not at all, or very seldom, and they breed but Weak and Tender Children.'[63] For Salmon the production of sickly children, that were perhaps likely to die soon after birth, was a form of barrenness. This perception of weak children and stillbirths may have endorsed the view that the initial conception needed to be strengthened. According to the humoural system, heat, vital spirits and nutrition could all affect the perfection of the initial conception and determine its likelihood of reaching parturition. These potent elements in generation could be supplemented by the use of provokers of lust. Thus it is possible that the anxiety expressed in medical texts about the fertility of the body and the accompanying promotion of aphrodisiacs was not only

---

[57] Peter Razzell and Christine Spence, 'The history of infant, child and adult mortality in London, 1550–1850', *London Journal* xxxii/3 (2007), 271–92 at pp. 271–2.
[58] Jones, 'Further evidence', 244.
[59] Ibid. 246.
[60] Ibid. 245; Razzell and Spence, 'The history of infant, child and adult mortality', 287.
[61] Galley, 'A never-ending succession of epidemics', 39.
[62] Ibid. 33, 37.
[63] William Salmon, *Systema medicinale, a compleat system of physick*, London 1686, 237.

influenced by the perception of widespread barrenness but also by an awareness of the precarious nature of early infant life.

Yet marital fertility and rates of child mortality were not universal topics of concern in early modern England. As medical and theological discourses were mutually dependent and influenced each other during this period, it is unsurprising that discussions about fertility in medical texts were implicitly and explicitly confined within the context of marriage. Therefore, although the medical texts confirm that aphrodisiacs were a widely understood category of medicaments, it was expected that these difficulties and the use of remedies to combat infertility and impotence were only experienced within the legitimate married sphere. The evidence presented in this book may therefore relate to a limited portion of early modern society.[64] Nevertheless, while the supposed use of sexual stimulants may only have been advocated in limited circumstances, the frequency of popular references to these substances suggests that they were widely understood by both married and unmarried men and women. The advertisement which opened this book shows that aphrodisiacs were also used in illicit circumstances.[65] Laura Gowing's work on illicit sexual activity has demonstrated that although everyday meals rarely featured in defamations of sexual sin, luxury food was described as prompting and sustaining sexual activity.[66] One of the cases that Gowing cites clearly shows one man using a well-known aphrodisiac, artichokes, in order to seduce the object of his affections: 'Peter Marsh had bin twice at her house and would have had her abroad with him to eate artichoks and drink wyne with him; And further that he the said Peter Marsh would have plucked her down into his lapp and would have putt his hands under her coate but that she would not suffer him.'[67] In this instance the sexual stimulants failed to arouse the man's intended partner, but it does show that aphrodisiacs were consumed, and given to others, in order to raise their lust and encourage them to engage in extra-marital sexual activity. The use of aphrodisiacs in this way has left few traces in the printed materials upon which this book is based. The works examined here instead clearly and consistently discussed aphrodisiacs in relation to marital duties and fertility. This strong connection may have limited the use of stimulants in illicit sexual encounters where conception was not the desired outcome. Yet it is plausible that cases like this were common, which would suggest, as this book will show occurred, that ideas about aphrodisiacs were adapted to fit individual circumstances. Although cases of seduction may be where modern

---

[64] A. M. Froide, 'Hidden women: rediscovering the single women of early modern England', *LPS* lxviii (2002), 26–41. Froide estimated that 34.2% of the population of Southampton were likely to be single women.

[65] McLaren, *Reproductive rituals*, 37.

[66] Laura Gowing, *Domestic dangers: women, words, and sex in early modern London*, Oxford 1996, 91.

[67] Ibid.

readers would expect to encounter the use of aphrodisiacs, there was another side to sexual stimulants that made their use much more common.

Religion, family, masculinity and sexuality

Fertility was a central aspect of early modern cultural ideals about marriage and sexuality. Under Christian teachings it was crucial that couples were able to engage in sexual intercourse and important that they were able produce offspring. The social place and roles of women were constructed around the idea of motherhood and the understanding of patriarchal, masculine sexuality was shaped by the desire to produce heirs, the physical manifestations of sexual potency and virility. These theological, and social, ideas permeated the understanding of barrenness and impotence presented in early modern medical treatises.

Theological discourse across the period emphasised the need for lust and sexuality to be confined within the legitimate boundaries of marriage. Principally procreation was deemed necessary in Genesis i.28 which stated that men and women should be fruitful and multiply. The implication of this was that sexuality was very often viewed through the prism of procreation. As Patricia Crawford has summarised, the Church viewed sexuality as a moral issue and so clerics taught the populace about morally acceptable, and unacceptable, sexual practices in printed works, sermons and informal teachings.[68] These teachings assumed that 'all sexuality should be heterosexual, genital and confined to marriage.'[69] The theological insistence on the reality of libidinous desires and their relationship to generation were reflected by medical writers. Helkiah Crooke highlighted the link between copulation and loving desire in his *Mikrokosmographia* (1615):

> that there might be a mutuall longing desire betweene the sexes to communicate one with another, and to conferre their stockes together for the propagation of mankinde, beside the ardor and heate of the spirits conteyned in their seeds, the parts of generation are so formed, that there is not onely a naturall instinct of copulation, but an appetite and earnest desire thereunto.[70]

The repetition of the theme of longing and desire suggests that this was an idea that medical men were eager to spread and disseminate. Many texts offered the suggestion that without pleasure and desire no man would enter into such a filthy and debauched situation. Similarly Crooke posited that no

---

[68] Patricia Crawford, *Blood, bodies and families in early modern England*, Harlow 2004, 55.
[69] Ibid.
[70] Helkiah Crooke, *Mikrokosmographia: a description of the body of man*, London 1615, 199.

woman would go through the ordeal of pregnancy and childbirth if it was not for the exquisite pleasure inherent in sexual intercourse.[71]

Beyond this it was also believed that marriage was the proper institution for the regulation of unbridled lusts. The marriage bed provided opportunities for the expression of sexuality and so negated the possibility of sinful acts such as fornication and adultery.[72] This was particularly important after the Reformation. Prior to the Reformation, Catholic doctrine had maintained that celibacy, especially monastic celibacy, allowed for a position of elevated spirituality. By contrast Protestantism attacked the ideal of celibacy and elevated the status of marriage to the ideal for almost everyone.[73] Martin Luther criticised celibacy not only because it prevented procreation, but also because he regarded sexual desire as natural and created by God.[74] Furthermore, marital sex was positive because it promoted affection between spouses and domestic harmony.[75] Erik Seeman has demonstrated how these Reformation ideas were inherited by English Protestants who praised marital sexuality as a legitimate outlet for natural urges.[76] Similarly Patricia Crawford has shown that William Perkins and William Gouge were proponents of both conceptive and sexually pleasing intercourse within marriage.[77] The medical discourse paralleled the theological. In *The secret miracles of nature* (1559) Lævinus Lemnius stated that 'Since this Passion is so forcible and so unruly that it can hardly be subdued (and but a few can bridle their passions) God granted unto man the use of the matrimonial bed, that he might be bounded thereby, and not defile themselves with wandring [sic] lust.'[78] In this context a successful marriage required pleasurable conjugal embraces, which could have been helped by recourse to sexual stimulants discussed by medical writers. It is likely that the prominence attributed to generative disorders at this time was heavily influenced by the importance of marital sexuality as advocated by churchmen.

More than theologians who referred to sexual drive, desire and pleasure in general terms, medical writers explored in detail the relationship between the reproductive organs/genitalia and pleasure. Jane Sharp in *The midwives book* (1671) frequently described parts of the sexed body, most notably the penis (or as it was often termed the yard), using the language of pleasure.

---

[71] Ibid. 200.

[72] James T. Johnson, 'English Puritan thought on the ends of marriage', *Church History* xxxviii/4 (1969), 429–36 at p. 429.

[73] Susan C. Karant-Nunn and Merry E. Wiesner-Hanks (eds), *Luther on women: a sourcebook*, Cambridge 2003, 137.

[74] Ibid.

[75] Ibid.

[76] Erik R. Seeman, '"It is better to marry than to burn": Anglo-American attitudes towards celibacy, 1600–1800', *JFH* xxiv/4 (1999), 397–419 at p. 400.

[77] Crawford, *Blood, bodies and family*, 56.

[78] Lævinus Lemnius, *The secret miracles of nature: in four books*, London [1559] 1658, 9.

She wrote that the sinews of the penis 'pass quite through the yard, and cause exceeding great delight when the Yard stands, and they prick forward in the action of venery'.[79] The use of descriptive terms such as this for all aspects of the sexed body reinforced the idea that healthy and pleasurable sexual behaviour was motivated by love and desire, emotions to be found within a marriage. The consequences of not feeling sexual desire for one's spouse were also explained. John Sadler's treatise *The sick womans private looking glasse* (1636) expressly related barrenness with a lack of love and desire. He explained to his readers that authors ascribed 'one maine cause of barrennesse to compeld copulation; as when parents enforce their daughters to have husbands contrary to their liking, therein marrying their bodies but not their hearts, and where there is a want of love, there for the most part is no conception'.[80] It is therefore apparent that reproductive capacity and conception were fundamentally and pervasively understood within a framework of love, desire and pleasure.

The legal sanctions for divorce were also affected by the theological teachings on marital sexuality. An inability to have sex and pay due benevolence constituted one of the four grounds for annulment in post-Reformation England, along with underage partners, prior contract of marriage, and marriage within the prohibited degrees.[81] Barrenness, however, was not an accepted reason for divorce; although some continental Protestants held that it was, England did not have a divorce law. Yet in some cases female infertility was considered grounds for separation. In the seventeenth century Dr Gilbert Burnet, a physician and bishop, was asked for his opinion, in reference to the fertility problems of King Charles and Queen Catherine, on the legality of dissolving a marriage because of infertility.[82] Although Burnet's comments were produced to aid the claims of those who wished the king and queen to divorce to ensure the stability of the monarchy and country, it is clear that he believed fertility was crucial to the viability and success of a marriage. Burnet expounded that,

> If therefore it be apparent that a Woman, either through the Situation and Disposition of her *Parts*, or some other Quality inherent in her *Matrix*, cannot *Conceive*; this being attested by Physicians, she is to be declared *Barren* ... A Woman being then found *Naturally Barren*, nothing of *Divorce* or *Polygamy*

---

[79] Sharp, *The midwives book*, 30.
[80] John Sadler, *The sick womans private looking glasse wherein methodically are handled all uterine affects, or diseases arising from ye wombe*, London 1636, 108–9.
[81] Martin Ingram, *Church courts, sex and marriage in England, 1570–1640*, Cambridge 1987, 145.
[82] John Macky, *Memoirs of the secret services of John Macky Esq.: during the reigns of King William, Queen Ann, and King George I*, London 1733, appendix II: 'Dr Gilbert Burnet's resolution of two important cases of conscience', p. xxiv.

is to be considered, but she is to be declared *incapable* of *Marriage*, as in the Case of *Frigidity* on the Man's Part: And so the *Marriage* is to be annulled.[83]

For Burnet, and those who sought his opinion, fertility was a key factor in dissolving a marriage, although this view never became law.[84] If a wife could not provide heirs and fulfil her motherly duties then she was incapable of marriage. Fertility was essential to a happy, secure and ordered marriage and society.

Particular prominence was given to male impotence in the legal status of a marriage, which had wider consequences for patriarchal authority and masculinity. In sixteenth-century France, as Pierre Darmon has shown, marriage was held to be a transaction, which impotent men entered into fraudulently knowing that they could not provide what was expected of them.[85] For many 'infertility threatened to belie the biblical pronouncements grounding the sacramental theory of marriage'.[86] This attitude was not limited to France; several scholars have demonstrated the existence of impotence trials for annulments and separations across early modern Europe.[87] Accusations of impotence consequently provided women with a way of pronouncing their husbands as ineffectual and weak, emasculating them in bodily and social terms. Moreover, if successful at trial, these accusations provided women with a means of escaping unhappy marriages.[88] Conversely, men who lost these cases could be barred from remarrying and had to live with the stigma of being sexually deficient.[89] When a man could not sexually satisfy his wife there was also always the possibility that she would transgress and break the patriarchal authority of her husband by cuckolding him. Anthony Fletcher has suggested that 'a husband's overriding imperative was to satisfy his wife in bed; the deepest shame was being called a cuckold'.[90]

The potential for men to be cuckolded became a fixation for writers of early modern erotic humour, particularly in ballads and chapbooks.[91] These

---

[83] Ibid. pp. xxvii–xxviii.

[84] In his description Burnet noted that this only applied to women of childbearing years; those who freely married older women were expected to live with their choice.

[85] Pierre Darmon, *Trial by impotence: virility and marriage in pre-revolutionary France*, trans. Paul Kegan, London 1985, 59.

[86] Ibid; Walter Stephens, 'Witches who steal penises: impotence and illusion in *Malleus maleficarum*', *Journal of Medieval and Early Modern Studies* xxviii/3 (1998), 495–516 at p. 499.

[87] Edward Behrend-Martinez, *Unfit for marriage: impotence spouses on trial in the Basque region of Spain, 1650–1750*, Reno 2007, 86.

[88] Ibid. 88–9.

[89] Ibid. 89.

[90] Anthony Fletcher, 'Manhood, the male body, courtship and the household in early modern England', *History* lxxxiv/275 (1999), 419–36 at p. 432.

[91] Roger Thompson, 'Popular reading and humour in Restoration England', *Journal of Popular Culture* ix/3 (1975), 653–71 at p. 666.

men were never treated with pity or compassion but were universally scorned as a subject for ridicule.[92] Ubiquitously symbolised by the wearing of horns, cuckolded men were blamed for the behaviour of scolding and adulterous wives, because they could not provide sexual satisfaction. In *The scolding wives vindication* the wife explained that she had no option but to cuff her husband around the ears because '*he would nothing do*'.[93] She further complained that 'Sometimes he'd give me a Kiss, and I wou'd return him two, But when he comes to farther Bliss *he nothing at all wou'd do*.'[94] Ballads such as this, not only represent the concerns felt by early modern society about the potential for social and marital disorder in the wake of impotence, but, as Roger Thompson has suggested, must also have reinforced and confirmed the virile masculinity of ordinary normal men.[95]

Ballads discussing the unenviable state of cuckolds may also have promoted the idea that aphrodisiacs could be one way to improve virility and satisfy a potentially adulterous wife. *The well-approved doctor: or an infallible cure for cuckolds* told the tale of 'a fine Doctor now new come to Town, Whose practice in physick had gain'd him renown, In curing of Cuckolds he had the best skill, By giving one Dose of his approved Pill'.[96] Although it is never made explicit what this medication is, it could plausibly have been an aphrodisiac. These were thought to enhance both sexual and generative abilities and thus allow a man to satisfy his wife's desires for intercourse and for offspring. This was not the only ballad to suggest that husbands could be sexually improved through the consumption of aphrodisiac substances. However, it was not always assumed that these medicaments would successfully cure impotence and infertility. Nonetheless it is apparent from ballads that seventeenth-century audiences readily accepted stories about male impotence and the effects that it could have on their lives, and that they also accepted the potential for using medical help to resolve this problem.

Beyond the adultery of their wives, male impotence and infertility was also connected to broader issues of patriarchy and manliness. Anthony Fletcher has examined the role of sexuality in the creation of masculinity and asserted that 'competitive adult manhood was defined in terms of sexual assertiveness and performance, learnt, practised and displayed'.[97] Potency and virility underpinned the ideals of masculinity and were an important part of developing into an adult male. Once manhood had been achieved a man's ability to engage in sex and have children underpinned both

---

[92] Ibid. See also McLaren, *Impotence*, 50–76.
[93] Anon., *The scolding wives vindication: or, An answer to the cuckold's complaint*, n.p. 1689.
[94] Ibid.
[95] Thompson, 'Popular reading and humour', 667.
[96] Anon., *The well-approved doctor: or, An infallible cure for cuckolds*, n.p. c. 1685–8).
[97] Fletcher, 'Manhood', 426.

marriage and the household.⁹⁸ Katie Barclay has argued that ballads and broadsheets suggest that women were willing to conform to their gender roles only if their husbands achieved ideal virile masculinity.⁹⁹ Thus impotence in popular culture represented the gendered struggle for authority: women would acquiesce to their passive feminine roles only if their husbands asserted their masculinity through sexual dominance and ability. As Angus McLaren has suggested, 'restoratives and sexual stimulants fulfilled social as well as sexual needs' because they restored manliness.¹⁰⁰ It was within this context that medical authors devoted such attention to the ways in which medicaments could enhance sexuality and potency. It was not only male vigour that was important to men's fulfilment of adult roles. Helen Berry and Elizabeth Foyster have investigated the concern surrounding 'childless men' at this time. They examined the role of fatherhood in creating male gender identity and patriarchy, and have shown that 'without children a married man's honour, reputation and credit were open to question'.¹⁰¹ They have argued that a weak male body was seen as weak both inside and outside of the bedroom and that this could have an impact on diverse aspects of social life including the ability to engage in politics and economic capacity.¹⁰² Simply put, an infertile or impotent man was seen as less of a man, unable to achieve true masculine or patriarchal authority. This was effectively highlighted in annulment cases where a marriage, a family and male patriarchy were dissolved because of the man's lack-lustre body. The inability to please his wife sexually was not only shaming but suggested a more general inability to manage his household and affairs. Berry and Foyster have demonstrated that this could be particularly traumatic with men exclaiming in 'a sighing sobbing tone of voice' their 'sorrow' at being unable to perform sexually.¹⁰³

However, scholars have debated the relative importance of fertility to married life. Angus McLaren stated in *Reproductive rituals* that children were highly prized as a sign of God's blessing, a source of security for the poor, and a proud sign of sexuality to men and a demonstration of maternal power to women.¹⁰⁴ Conversely, Alan Macfarlane has argued that these reasons were not important to early modern parents who instead wanted children for their

---

[98] Ibid. 427.
[99] Katie Barclay, '"And four years space, being man and wife, they loveingly agreed": balladry and early modern understanding of marriage', in Elizabeth Ewan and Janay Nugent (eds), *Finding the family in medieval and early modern Scotland*, Aldershot 2008, 23–33 at p. 31.
[100] McLaren, *Impotence*, 57–8.
[101] Berry and Foyster, 'Childless men', 159, 178.
[102] Ibid. 178–9.
[103] Ibid. 180.
[104] McLaren, *Reproductive rituals*, 32.

own psychological gratification.¹⁰⁵ In contrast to McLaren, he has argued that the religious motivation to have children was 'singularly weak' and that for every person who was motivated by religion 'there were a hundred swayed by lust'.¹⁰⁶ While there may have been many pregnancies that occurred as the result of lustful encounters, viewing lust in this way does not acknowledge the intimate connection that existed between sexual desire and procreation in the early modern mind-set. Macfarlane draws heavily on the ideas of Malthus and contrasts Christianity's ideas about fertility with Hindu, Muslim and Confucian concerns and concludes that in comparison there was very little pressure to conceive and have children in the Christian religion.¹⁰⁷ So although he believed that children were seen as a blessing, they were not seen as a religious imperative. Macfarlane similarly argued that children in the early modern period were not considered as a way of increasing social prestige and status, but rather that numerous children were seen as a financial burden.¹⁰⁸ This interpretation is again problematic as it fails to allow for society to view moderate fertility as a blessing but simultaneously express concern about voracious fertility. Scholars have since returned to McLaren's original assessment of the importance, both social and religious, of fertility. Oren-Magidor has shown that descriptions and understandings of infertility were intimately bound to religious and moral ideas, and that being infertile could certainly damage social status. Similarly Laura Gowing has emphasised how barren women and infertile/impotent men were liable to the scorn and ridicule of their neighbours.¹⁰⁹ Moreover, is clear that both popular and medical literature viewed barrenness in biblical and spiritual terms; it was inflicted and remedied by God.

The specific concerns for fertility within a marriage also reflected broader anxieties about sterility and depopulation, particularly amongst the aristocracy. At the very top of society there were concerns about the dynastic stability of the monarchy.¹¹⁰ Across the period, and across Europe, several monarchs struggled to father a child. For example, Catherine of Braganza, consort to Charles II and queen of England, failed to conceive any children and was reported to suffer from dysfunctional uterine bleeding.¹¹¹ Catherine was evidently concerned about this and visited the spas at Tunbridge Wells

---

¹⁰⁵ Alan Macfarlane, *Marriage and love in England: modes of reproduction, 1300–1840*, Oxford 1986, 51.

¹⁰⁶ Ibid. 57.

¹⁰⁷ Ibid. 58.

¹⁰⁸ Ibid. 60.

¹⁰⁹ Laura Gowing, *Common bodies: women, touch, and power in seventeenth century England*, New Haven–London 2003, 115.

¹¹⁰ Mary Fissell, *Vernacular bodies: the politics of reproduction in early modern England*, Oxford 2004, 196.

¹¹¹ ODNB, *s.v.* 'Catherine', accessed 2 Aug. 2013.

and Bath in an effort to cure her barrenness.[112] There was also concern amongst eighteenth-century writers, as Robin Ganev has stressed, that the English were not producing enough healthy children to defend the nation.[113] These concerns also tied into wider ideas about sexuality as fears were expressed that the aristocracy were less fertile than the lower classes. Writers often contrasted the vigorous and virile sexuality of the agricultural, rural, classes and the 'impotent nobility, whose sexuality was debilitated by urban luxury'.[114] These stereotypes existed throughout the period in the medical literature: William Buchan wrote in 1772 that 'it is very certain that high living vitiates the humours, and prevents fecundity'.[115] He further asserted that, in line with Ganev's interpretation of eighteenth-century discourse on fertility, 'we seldom find a barren woman among the labouring poor, while nothing is more common amongst the rich and affluent'.[116] Ganev argued that 'every aspect of city life was imagined to be bad for one's sex drive' and that it was believed that the upper classes substituted other luxuries for sexual pleasure and so had no need of intercourse.[117] It was perhaps these anxieties about the upper classes that caused medical writers to continue discussing impotence, barrenness and sexual stimulants in such detail even as the fertility upswings suggested by demographers began to make their impact felt on population levels.

What is clear from discussions about religion and the family, masculinity and sexuality, is that sexual pleasure, ability and potency were central to the maintenance of an ordered and stable society. Infertility threatened the microcosm of the home. It was thus imperative that the medical discourse acknowledged, explained and described remedies designed to counter reproductive failure.

One of the central premises of this book is that a certain broad understanding of sex, generation and aphrodisiacs was shared by a large proportion of the populace. This is shown by drawing upon a diverse collection of printed and manuscript materials which contain discussions of aphrodisiacs and their qualities. Chapter 1 introduces these genres and demonstrates that early modern society was one that was highly informed about the body and medicine. Men and women were encouraged to understand their own constitutions and health and to work actively to maintain their health or recover it when they fell ill.

---

[112] Ibid.
[113] Robin Ganev, 'Milkmaids, ploughmen, and sex in eighteenth-century Britain', *Journal of the History of Sexuality* xvi/1 (2007), 40–67 at p. 46.
[114] Ibid 42.
[115] William Buchan, *Domestic medicine: or, A treatise on the prevention and cure of diseases by regimen and simple medicine*, London 1772, 667.
[116] Ibid.
[117] Ganev, 'Milkmaids, ploughmen, and sex', 43, 45.

When faced with bouts of ill health men and women became active and well-informed customers and consumers in a complex and competitive medical marketplace. To treat infertility they sought advice from the knowledge recorded in manuscript collections, gathered information from relatives and friends and bought the services of a range of medical practitioners. Understanding how men and women gained medical knowledge and medical care thus helps us to understand that even though the majority of this book draws upon the intellectual discourses about fertility and aphrodisiacs found in printed works, it can be assumed that this knowledge was never simply a passive element of society. It is plausible that men and women when faced with infertility and impotence did in fact seek out, purchase and consume the aphrodisiacs with which they were familiar.

Chapter 2 scrutinises the understanding of the reproductive and infertile bodies that was propounded in the medical treatises available across the sixteenth, seventeenth and eighteenth centuries. Sexual desire and pleasure were considered crucial for the body to be fertile. Moreover, there were many ways in which medical writers believed that the reproductive system could be damaged and distempered. This created scope for many different types of substances to be thought of as aphrodisiacs. The understanding of infertility, and its treatment, was however influenced by the ways in which medical writers understood sex and gender. This chapter demonstrates that across the early modern period the language of infertility became increasingly sex/gender-specific. Despite this, however, the continued acceptance of similarities between the two body types meant that the aetiologies of male and female infertility were thought to be the same.

The centrality of sexual desire and pleasure to conception is further explored in chapter 3, which examines the ways in which medical writers and the wider populace understood the effects of aphrodisiacs. Medical writers believed that some were 'hindered very much for want of desire to be acquainted with Venus' and so were infertile.[118] Consequently the first way in which sexual stimulants were thought to cure infertility was by encouraging men and women to engage in sexual activity. Yet more than this, medical writers explained in detail that aphrodisiac substances improved the ability of the reproductive body to experience sexual pleasure, which was requisite for the release of seed to allow for conception. They also improved the temperature and seed production of the generative organs making them more fertile. Medical writers did not, though, advocate stimulating substances without questioning their effects. Those that were found to be ineffective, particularly those that did not improve fertility as well as sexual drive, were critiqued and dismissed.

Not all instances of infertility and impotence were thought to be the

---

[118] Jakob Rueff, *The expert midwife: or, An excellent and most necessary treatise of the generation and birth of man*, London 1637, 55–61.

result of straightforward physical ailments: it was also believed that witchcraft could be utilised to maliciously inflict impotence and infertility upon individuals and couples. Despite the increasing scepticism that witchcraft was a corporeal reality that was developing across the early modern period, Angus McLaren has argued that throughout the seventeenth century men and women in this situation focused upon magical and ritualistic cures.[119] Conversely, in chapter 4 it will be argued that medical treatises, in line with the religious rejection of ritualistic responses, throughout the period, although including some ritualistic and sympathetic cures, focused on the use of natural remedies and in particular the use of aphrodisiacs in order to restore the fertility and sexual vigour of those who had been bewitched.

Early modern medical writers viewed barrenness as an overall inability to have children. In particular there were two elements of women's reproductive health that had to be managed in order to ensure their fertility. The absence of menstruation was considered to be an important cause of female infertility. Consequently women were encouraged to use remedies that provoked menstrual bleeding in order to restore their fertility. These drugs have often been interpreted as covert means of aborting an unwanted foetus by removing blockages and stimulating bleeding. Yet, as chapter 5 will demonstrate, by examining the similarities between emmenagogues and aphrodisiacs, and by detailing the clear presence of sexual stimulants in compound remedies of this nature, it is apparent that these remedies were also a part of regimes designed to promote fertility. Secondly, it was necessary for a woman to carry a child to term, and so chapter 5 also examines whether or not the consumption of aphrodisiacs was thought to help in maintaining a healthy pregnancy. It suggests that although a context existed within which aphrodisiacs could have been used for this purpose, medical writers were reluctant to do so. The belief that sexual intercourse, and excessive sexual stimulation, could result in miscarriage prevented authors from advocating the full range of stimulants in this way.

Aphrodisiacs did more than just provoke lust and they were more than just sexual curiosities; they worked in ways that are unfamiliar to modern readers and were a crucial element in the struggle for fertility. As such they ask us to reconsider preconceived notions about the distinctive nature of the reproductive and sexual bodies.

---

[119] McLaren, *Impotence*, 52.

1

Texts, Readers and Markets

In *The ten pleasures of marriage* (1682) a young woman worried that she had been married three months and was yet to get pregnant. She began to gossip with her neighbours and sought their advice about the virility and sexual abilities of her husband:

> Whosoever she speaks with every one pities her, and gives her their advice: And the best sort will at the least say to her, I would oftentimes treat my husband with such sort of spices as were good for my self, *viz*. Oisters, Egs, Coxcombs, sweet breads, Lam-stones, Caveer [sic], &c. and counsell him every morning to go to the Coffe-house [sic] and drink some Chocolate.[1]

In this humorous tale of the difficulties of marriage, the author makes it clear that knowledge about aphrodisiacs, good for both the husband and the wife, is part of women's everyday sexual and medical knowledge. This book will demonstrate that this indeed was the case, and that a shared understanding of what foods, and other substances, were aphrodisiacs and how they functioned could be found in a variety of printed and manuscript sources from 1550 to 1780.

To do so it will use a broad survey of printed medical literature, including general treatises and those specialising in generation, botanical texts, popular and ephemeral literature, medical advertisements and manuscript recipe books. This is an approach to the study of cultural ideas about the body that has already been successfully utilised by scholars like Bethan Hindson.[2] Although the sources used in this book do not always provide directly comparable evidence, and even though this approach runs the risk of decontextualising and ignoring the specific traditions of each source genre, the benefits of this approach more than compensate for these problems. Comparing a range of source material provides a compelling overview of the ways in which aphrodisiacs were understood in this period. The many points of intersection between these genres, and the ways in which they disagree, help to build a clear yet nuanced picture of how men and women perceived sexual stimulation through food and medicine. As *The ten pleasures of marriage* shows, descriptions of aphrodisiacs and suggestions about their function could be

---

[1] A. Marsh, *The ten pleasures of marriage relating all the delights and contentments that are mask'd under the bands of matrimony*, London 1682, 77.
[2] Bethan Hindson, 'Attitudes towards menstruation and menstrual blood in Elizabethan England', *JSH* xliii/1 (2009), 89–114.

found in a range of non-medical and popular literature. The presence of aphrodisiacs in works like this one, as well as in ballads and erotic literature, illustrates that the ideas presented in medical texts were not confined to the medical discourse, but were a part of the sexual and reproductive knowledge of the wider populace. This book also closely considers the importance of gender in the descriptions of aphrodisiacs in medical texts. Works such as the *The ten pleasures of marriage* allow us to ask whether common understandings of aphrodisiacs were also 'sexed': how far were certain stimulants thought to be relevant only to the male or only to the female body? Although the non-medical texts do not often form the basis of the arguments, they illuminate the ways in which medical ideas interacted with broader cultural ideals of social and gender relationships and behaviours.

Although this book is predominantly about the ways in which men and women understood aphrodisiacs and their functions, the sources used here can also hint at possible medical practice. It is not suggested that men and women always utilised aphrodisiacs when they believed themselves to be infertile, but simply that the ubiquity of their presence in medical texts and other genres suggests that they were likely to have been used and consumed. Printed treatises, particularly medical ones, did not simply represent theoretical knowledge but were often actively read by early modern men and women to find useful information that could be practically applied to their own lives. It is important therefore to consider in more detail book production and reading at this time. This chapter will introduce these sources and discuss the ways in which readers engaged with the medical knowledge that they found in such texts. It will also explore the various means by which, if they so desired, early modern men and women could purchase, produce and consume sexual stimulants.

Texts and readers

Medical texts in early modern England were a heterogeneous genre. Works were still produced and circulated in manuscript form, while the upsurge in the production of printed medical texts from around 1550 greatly increased the number and variety of texts available.[3] However, until the early seventeenth century the majority of medical works were produced in the *lingua franca* of medical knowledge, Latin.[4] During the seventeenth century the numbers of medical works produced in English increased. In particular the closure of the Star Chamber in 1641 removed the government's means of

---

[3] Irma Taavitsainen, Peter Murray Jones, Paivi Pahta, Turo Hiltunen, Ville Marttila, Maura Rtia, Carla Suhr and Jukka Tyrkko, 'Medical texts in 1500–1700 and the corpus of early modern English medical texts', in Irma Taavitsainen and Paivi Pahta (eds), *Medical writing in early modern English*, Cambridge 2011, 9–25 at pp. 9–10.
[4] Ibid. 12.

conducting censorship trials and allowed for a flourishing trade in vernacular printed materials on a variety of subjects.[5] Medical advice literature and medical treatises ranging from cheap palm-sized books to costly folios, particularly those exploring the great mystery of generation, were increasingly popular. The production of these texts was fostered by the influence of radicals who railed against the medical elitism that they perceived in the Royal College of Physicians and in Latin works.[6] Between 1649 and 1699, 282 books on medical-chemical and astrological themes alone were registered with the Stationers' Company.[7] Book production, including medical literature, was concentrated in London, Cambridge and Oxford, although provincial presses were also created in Exeter, Newcastle, York and Worcester. The provincial book trade was consequently focused on the distribution of texts through booksellers and itinerant sellers, including pedlars and chapmen. By the 1580s bookselling in provincial towns was firmly established.[8]

Many of the medical texts published during this period were not written by English physicians, surgeons or anatomists. They were translations or republications of works originally written on the continent by European medical practitioners, physicians and medical professors. In particular few original works of anatomy were produced in England, because dissection interfered with a body's readiness for the final judgement. It was therefore important that English medical practitioners had access to the works of continental anatomists.[9] The publication of medical works in Latin created a shared European culture of medicine. England was not isolated in terms of medical developments and understanding: it was a part of the broader culture of medical enquiry, innovation and learning that was practised in universities across Europe. The surgeon who translated the French surgical treatise of Henri-François Le Dran implored his readers to accept the knowledge that it contained regardless of its country of origin:

> *I hope the Performance being the Product of a foreign Country, will be no Objection to it. Arts and Sciences are cultivated with the View of a general Benefit to our Fellow Creatures; and though we should have a political Objection to any Nation, does it follow that we should not embrace the Sciences of that Nation for our own*

---

[5] Ibid. 14.

[6] Gowing, *Common bodies*, 17.

[7] Mary Rhinelander McCarl, 'Publishing the works of Nicholas Culpeper, astrological herbalist and translator of Latin medical works in seventeenth-century London', *Canadian Bulletin of Medical History* xiii/2 (1996), 225–76 at p. 230.

[8] John Barnard and Maureen Bell, 'The English provinces', in John Barnard and D. F. McKenzie (eds), *The Cambridge history of the book in Britain, IV: 1557–1695*, Cambridge 2002, 665–86 at pp. 666–7, 673.

[9] Elizabeth Lane Furdell, *Publishing and medicine in early modern England*, New York 2002, 50.

Advantage? I hope we are too much Englishmen *to imagine we cannot improve by them, since they are so generous as to acknowledge they have improved by us.*[10]

These European texts also connected with the medical culture of the new world as European printing occupied a central position in the commercial book markets of colonial America.[11] The translation of these works into the vernacular increased their accessibility and their readership. Foreign works were an integral part of British medical knowledge as medical writers, practitioners and consumers all participated in a shared European medical culture.

As the major expansion in medical printing occurred during the Civil War it is plausible to assume that some of the two hundred printers and sellers who handled medical texts were motivated by religion and politics.[12] Yet Elizabeth Lane Furdell has suggested that while the Puritan-parliamentary coalition wanted to see the production of medical knowledge in the vernacular political influence on medical publishing was not strong.[13] Instead there was a variety of writers, publishers and sellers producing works from all sides of the political and religious spectrum.[14] These publishers were willing to produce and sell medical works by authors diametrically opposed in belief and status, including Galenic, Helmontian and Paracelsian works.[15] Hence Furdell concluded that the only discernible motivation in the publication of medical texts was profit.[16] The drive for profit was particularly apparent in those who published and sold texts attributed to and written by Nicholas Culpeper, an apothecary who railed against the elitism of the Royal College of Physicians and the printing of medical knowledge in Latin and so published numerous medical treatises in English. The publishers Peter Cole and Nathaniel Brooks, and others, used printed prefaces and book advertisements placed in Culpeper's works to persuade buyers to purchase further volumes from their lists.[17] The 1662 edition of *The directory for midwives* included four pages of other works produced by Cole in the front of the book and a further two and a half pages listing other works of Culpeper at the back.[18] They hoped that the association with Culpeper's name would

---

[10] Henri-François le Dran, *Observations in surgery: containing one hundred and fifteen different cases*, London 1739, p. vi.

[11] Hugh Amory, 'British books abroad: the American colonies', in Barnard and McKenzie, *Cambridge history of the book*, iv. 744–52 at p. 745; James Raven, *The business of books: booksellers and the English book trade, 1450–1850*, New Haven– London 2007, 144.

[12] Furdell, *Publishing and medicine*, 49.

[13] Ibid. 59.

[14] Ibid. 70.

[15] Ibid. 71–3.

[16] Ibid. 73.

[17] McCarl, 'Publishing the works of Nicholas Culpeper', 226.

[18] Culpeper, *Culpeper's directory for midwives* (1662 edn), A3r–A4v, 270–2.

give them greater appeal.[19] Mary Rhinelander McCarl has explained that after 1660 many of Culpeper's translations were still published, now aimed at poorer and less educated readers, even though they were thought to be somewhat outdated.[20] Although they did not contain the latest medical theories, publishers still perceived that his works had an audience and would sell. Both Furdell and McCarl concluded that politics and religion had little to do with the production and sale of medical texts. Instead profit drove the commissioning, publishing and printing of these works during the early modern period.

The drive for profit displayed by book sellers was reflected in the cost of medical treatises. Sachiko Kusukawa has demonstrated that large scholarly tomes could be very expensive, with the cost of the paper accounting for most of the price.[21] Treatises that included images, such as pictures of plants or dissection diagrams, were considerably more expensive, as much as double the price, for a comparable book.[22] The cost of such items obviously restricted their sale to the wealthy or to universities where they were used in medical education. Yet not all book purchasers bought their items new. Mary Fissell has shown that numerous medical texts were sold at auction for lower prices and so circulated more widely.[23] Purchasing a work through the second-hand trade made them available to a wider cross-section of society.[24] It also ensured that medical treatises had a long shelf-life, which helped to create a medical culture where changes of orthodoxy were slow to occur, and where both new and old ideas could be discussed and debated concurrently.

The analysis in this book is predicated on the ideas that medical treatises of various kinds were relatively widely accessed, and that reading a book in the early modern period was not a passive activity. Scholars have estimated that a substantial proportion of the early modern population was able to read. Margaret Spufford has argued that many children were equipped with a rudimentary knowledge of reading in the home, while boys from yeoman, husbandman and labouring backgrounds were often sent to school to learn how to read.[25] She has concluded that there was likely a 30 per

---

[19] McCarl, 'Publishing the works of Nicholas Culpeper', 230.

[20] Ibid. 252.

[21] Sachiko Kusukawa, *Picturing the book of nature: image, text, and argument in sixteenth-century human anatomy and medical botany*, Chicago 2012, 50.

[22] Ibid.

[23] Mary Fissell, 'The marketplace of print', in Mark S. R. Jenner and Patrick Wallis (eds), *Medicine and the market in England and its colonies, c. 1450–1850*, Basingstoke 2007, 108–32 at p. 112. See also Tessa Watt, *Cheap print and popular piety, 1550–1640*, Cambridge 1991, introduction.

[24] Fissell, 'The marketplace of print, 112.

[25] Margaret Spufford, 'First steps in literacy: the reading and writing experiences of the humblest seventeenth century spiritual autobiographers', *Social History* iv/3 (1979), 407–35 at pp. 433, 435, 410–12.

cent male readership and an unknown female readership of small books and popular ephemera after the 1660s.[26] Access to literate culture was not only restricted to those who could read: Roger Chartier and Tessa Watt have argued that reading aloud was central to early modern reading practices and that this practice disseminated the knowledge contained in printed works to a diverse audience who could not afford the works themselves or could not read them.[27] Stephen Dobranski has shown that consumers of print materials made texts meaningful to themselves and appropriated the knowledge in books for their own ends.[28] In the case of medical works and herbals, readers recorded potentially useful remedies and used the medical knowledge that they acquired to assist them in obtaining medical care. Indeed, one author in a collection of culinary and medical recipes owned by Mary Glover in 1688 listed the virtues of certain herbs according to Culpeper, which suggests that they actively accumulated knowledge from printed works.[29] Dobranski has also suggested that many saw writing and reading as a collaborative process, where authors were given credence and authority by the reception of their book.[30] For example the preface to William Harvey's *Anatomical exercitations* explained that the work needed a friendly reader to make his ideas meaningful and influential.[31] The collaborative nature of printed works was influenced by the humanist traditions of learning which advocated reading works comparatively and historically to transform the text into something useful which could be applied to the pursuit of knowledge.[32] This tradition informed the practice of keeping a commonplace book where useful information from reading, and discussions with friends, was recorded to create a new volume of knowledge specific to individual needs. This was then further developed into the practice of collecting, testing and recording culinary and medical recipes from medical texts, friends and experimentation.

Printed and manuscript texts were thus interconnected sources of medical knowledge at this time. Readers used printed medical treatises to form opinions on, record, and possibly use, the recipes that they came across. Michael Hunter and Annabel Gregory have shown that Samuel Jeake, a seventeenth-century merchant and astrologer, owned and read numerous medical texts including Culpeper's translation of Lazarus Riverius' *Practice*

---

[26] Idem, *Small books and pleasant histories: popular fiction and its readership in seventeenth-century England*, Cambridge 1981, 22.

[27] Roger Chartier, *The order of books: readers, authors, and libraries in Europe between the fourteenth and eighteenth centuries*, Cambridge 1994, 19–20; Watt, *Cheap print*, 7–8.

[28] Stephen Dobranski, *Readers and authorship in early modern England*, Cambridge 2005, 22.

[29] BL, MS Add. 57944, fo. 10v.

[30] Dobranski, *Readers and authorship*, 22, 51.

[31] Ibid. 51.

[32] Ibid. 25.

of physick (1655).³³ Jeake's medical reading encompassed works which challenged Galenic orthodoxy as well as studies by pioneering contemporaries like William Harvey and Thomas Bartholin.³⁴ Like Mary Glover's family, Philip Frith, a member of Jeake's social circle, kept a commonplace book which recorded medical lore and recipes.³⁵ This acquired knowledge was then used in their interactions with physicians and medical practitioners: patients shaped their enquiries and vocabulary of illness from these works and then expressed opinions, expectations and criticisms of medications that they were prescribed.³⁶ The collection of medical knowledge was not a gendered practice – both men and women actively engaged with medical treatises – although women's practices could be circumscribed by the cultural norms of silence and modesty.³⁷ However, these concerns do not appear to have drastically affected women's access to vernacular medical texts or their desire to demonstrate the knowledge that they acquired: Elizabeth Hunt wrote defiantly inside a volume of *Culpeper's directory for midwives* that it was 'hers not his' (in reference to her husband).³⁸ Moreover, as the quotation that opened this chapter suggested, it was expected that some women would have knowledge about sexual matters.

It was not only through keeping collections of recipes that men and women actively engaged with medical treatises. Michael Solomon has shown that in Spain throughout the medieval and early modern periods medical books were used as a physical representation or substitution for an absent physician; they were able to do this because they claimed to allow ordinary men and women to act autonomously from a practising physician.³⁹ Traditionally, Solomon argued, tension existed between the ways in which physicians understood disease, through Latinate culture, and how patients understood illness through pain and bodily dysfunction.⁴⁰ Similarly, in England, Andrew Wear has shown that while many accepted that lay (non-medical) persons understood the symptoms of illness and could make crude diagnoses, they

---

³³ Michael Hunter and Annabel Gregory (eds), *An astrological diary of the seventeenth century: Samuel Jeake of Rye, 1652–1699*, Oxford 1988, 46; *ODNB*, *s.v.* 'Samuel Jeake', accessed 28 Mar. 10.

³⁴ Hunger and Gregory, *An astrological diary*, 46–7.

³⁵ Ibid. 53.

³⁶ Deborah Harkness, '*Nosce te ipsum*: curiosity, the humoural body and the culture of therapeutics in late sixteenth- and early seventeenth-century England', in R. J. W. Evans and Alexander Marr (eds), *Curiosity and wonder from the Renaissance to the Enlightenment*, Aldershot 2006, 171–92 at pp. 179, 181.

³⁷ Heidi Brayman Hackel has also suggested that women's reading could be trivialised as diversions interchangeable with needlework or lapdogs: *Reading material in early modern England: print, gender and literacy*, Cambridge 2005, 207.

³⁸ Ibid. 214–15.

³⁹ Michael Solomon, *Fictions of well-being: sickly readers and vernacular medical writing in late medieval and early modern Spain*, Philadelphia–Oxford 2010, 26–9.

⁴⁰ Ibid. 35.

were not able to interpret the signs of the body to identify accurately the underlying cause of the disease.[41] In this context patients could use a vernacular text in order to create an imagined middle ground where the necessary interaction between patient and physician might take place.[42]

Finally, it is worth considering not just that these printed treatises provided medical and sexual knowledge to a diverse audience, but also that the information that they portrayed changed and developed throughout the period. New ideas about anatomy, the body and medicine were not instantly accepted and older ideas that were increasingly subject to criticism were not immediately discarded in the printed medical literature. It was often the case that new ideas were incorporated into the existing corpus of knowledge and only gradually replaced what were then understood to be 'erroneous' assertions. Several medical writers adopted an approach that best showed off their learning and knowledge, which involved including a range of varying opinions of a given topic, both old and new, and either letting the reader decide which was the most convincing or eventually siding with one theory over another. For example, while describing the form and function of the testicles, the 1663 edition of the *Bartholinus anatomy* explained to readers that Hippocrates had said that the seed (sperm) from the left testicle produced girls, while that from the right produced boys.[43] The author included a description of why this was the case, even though he went on to say 'but I am not of [the] Opinion, that wenches are alwaies [sic] begotten by the left Stone' and then to explain in detail why this was incorrect.[44]

As in the *Bartholinus anatomy*, some authors did argue in favour of newer ideas, but we cannot be certain that their readers accepted their opinions. Instead they may have favoured the older, more familiar, theories that they found in these works. Similarly the popularity of the longstanding Galenic, Hippocratic and Aristotelian theories of generation encouraged writers who wanted to attract a broad vernacular audience to continue to perpetuate these older ideas. As Patricia Crawford has summarised, early modern medical texts

> range from original contributions to rehashes of old ideas, for there is no clear line of progress in medical knowledge during the seventeenth century. It took time for important discoveries to be accepted, and many physicians still tried to fit new ideas into the framework of the ancient classical medical theories.[45]

---

[41] Andrew Wear, *Knowledge and practice in English medicine, 1550–1680*, Cambridge 2000, 111–12.

[42] Solomon, *Fictions of well-being*, 35.

[43] Thomas Bartholin, *Bartholinus anatomy; made from the precepts of his father, and from the observations of all modern anatomists; together with his own*, London 1663, 55.

[44] Ibid.

[45] Crawford, *Blood, bodies and families*, 20.

As Crawford suggests, one reason why older ideas continued to be perpetuated was because many medical treatises drew heavily upon existing works, in some cases plagiarising sections of text verbatim. This is particularly evident in midwifery manuals: Peter Chamberlain's work, *Dr. Chamberlain's midwifes practice*, was used by Jane Sharp to create *The midwives book* and Lævinus Lemnius' tracts were reused by the anonymous author of the popular *Aristotle's master-piece*.[46] Several treatises were also reprinted in later centuries, like Thomas Raynalde's *Birth of mankind* which was available from 1540 to 1654, and *Aristotle's master-piece*, which was published, as a complete treatise, in 1684 and went through approximately 130 editions by 1800.[47] Thus the book trade comprised a mixture of books, some of which were original pieces incorporating new ideas and others that were either new editions of old works or old treatises re-worked into new publications. The relative dominance of traditional theories of generation created substantial continuity in the aphrodisiacs that were discussed and recommended by medical writers and the wider populace throughout the sixteenth, seventeenth and eighteenth centuries.

Medical texts were not the only source of information about sexual stimulants. Botanical works and herbals provided details about plants, both English and foreign; what they looked like, when they grew, flowered and seeded, and what medicinal properties they had. The interest in botany and botanical publishing increased substantially in the second half of the sixteenth century.[48] Concurrently the scholarly respect afforded to the study of plants increased. Traditionally physicians had had little to do with plants before they were processed into medicines. However, in the sixteenth century they were increasingly criticised for their ignorance in this area.[49] The popularity of herbals was short-lived; by the mid-seventeenth century the publication of such works had significantly declined and they were gradually replaced by botanical encyclopaedias.[50] These treatises were part of the broader culture of collecting knowledge.[51] Kusukawa has described how Conrad Gessner amassed a wealth of knowledge about plants including notes and images which functioned as a pictorial commonplace, which he intended to publish as a *Historia planatarum*.[52] Botanical treatises were similar to manuscript

---

[46] Fissell, *Vernacular bodies*, 198–9.

[47] Elaine Hobby (ed.), *The birth of mankind: otherwise named, the woman's book*, Farnham 2009, p. xv; I am grateful to Mary Fissell for sharing information on the number of editions of the *Master-piece*.

[48] Leah Knight, *Of books and botany in early modern England: sixteenth-century plants and print culture*, Farnham 2009, 6; Brent Elliott, 'The world of the Renaissance herbal', *Renaissance Studies* xxv/1 (2011), 24–41.

[49] Knight, *Of books and botany*, 16.

[50] Elliott, 'The world of the Renaissance herbal', 39

[51] Knight, *Of books and botany*, 4.

[52] Kusukawa, *Picturing the book of nature*, 139–61.

recipe collections in that they collected and presented useful knowledge about the natural world.

One of the most frequently referenced herbals in this work is John Gerard's *Generall historie of plantes*, first published in 1597. The reason for its inclusion rather than others is not only its comprehensiveness, but also that Gerard had a medical background. He was trained as a barber-surgeon before acting as curator of the physic garden created by the Royal College of Physicians.[53] His work therefore demonstrates an understanding of the medical virtues of plants that, it can be assumed, was relatively consistent with the medical knowledge of the College, and of other practitioners, at the time. Indeed, William Drage, an apothecary in Hitchin, stated, in *Physical experiments* (1668), of his own practice that 'I have chiefly trusted to Simples commended by *Gerards* and other Herbals, for they were experienced good in such Distempers they are praised'.[54] Gerard's text, like medical texts, borrowed heavily from earlier works, including William Turner's herbal (part I published in 1551 and part II in 1562). Turner, as a trained physician, was also interested in the medical properties of plants. Many of these herbals were thus originally produced by academically trained medical men as a scholarly endeavour aimed at their contemporaries.[55] Even so, the information that they contained was still relevant and of interest to the wider populace; consequently these treatises were often reshaped and reprinted in forms that made them accessible to a broader audience.[56]

As has been suggested, knowledge from both medical works and herbals was incorporated into manuscript recipe collections. Early investigations into these collections suggested that their creation and compilation was a gendered practice, particularly as women were described as the primary healers within a household. However, Elaine Leong has since emphasised that these collections were kept by men and women, and more commonly collectively by families. As bequests these collections moved through the generations and were formed of and expanded by knowledge gathered through household, family and kinship.[57] These collections reflect the desire to possess tangible forms of health care provision and, to a limited extent, demonstrate popular medical practice. Recipe books developed out of the medieval tradition of commonplace books, which brought together collections of proverbs, recipes and other useful selections from a range of sources.[58] The practice

---

[53] ODNB, s.v. 'John Gerard', accessed 17 Apr. 2013.

[54] William Drage, *Physical experiments: being a plain description of the causes, signes, and cures of most diseases incident to the body of man*, London 1668, 42.

[55] Knight, *Of books and botany*, 22.

[56] Ibid.

[57] Elaine Leong, 'Collecting knowledge for the family: recipes, gender and practical knowledge in the early modern English household', *Centaurus* lv/2 (2013), 81–103 at p. 84.

[58] Catherine Field, '"Many hands hands": writing the self in early modern women's

of keeping these books was influenced by the humanist reading and writing practices of collecting, organising and generating specialised knowledge in books structured thematically by topic.[59] Although these collections were designed to contain useful information, to a modern reader it can appear that they lack the information requisite to cure illness. In many cases practical information about the strength or amounts of ingredients used in medical recipes is absent.[60] In other recipes the author is not explicit about how the ingredients should be combined. This was because it was expected that those compiling these works would gather this information orally or would know the strengths and quantities of herbs needed and so this information was left to the discretion of the cook. Similarly recipe books were experimental in nature: it was assumed that women, and men, would produce these remedies, using their own knowledge, refining them until they were satisfied with the overall efficacy of the remedy and would adapt them to suit the temperament and condition of different patients.[61] Compilers and producers of medicines were expected to build up their knowledge through a working system of testing, which can in many cases be seen in the annotations and crossings out that adorn many recipe collections. Recipes were not simply accepted because they existed in a collection; each new owner would evaluate and test the remedy, crossing out those that were no longer considered effective.[62] Not all the information recorded in these texts was experimental though. In several collections remedies were attributed to printed sources such as those by William Salmon or to doctors and medical practitioners.[63] Recipes were also recorded that had been provided by physicians. Yet this does not reveal a solely top-down process of knowledge development; popular medical practice also informed and influenced what medical writers incorporated into their treatises. Recipe collections were often passed down through female lines and many include recipes written in many different hands. They thus represent knowledge accumulated and refined over time rather than a snapshot of medical understanding at any one point. This can particularly be seen where subsequent owners have gone through and crossed out the recipes of their predecessors that were now considered obsolete or ineffective.

Several recipe collections included remedies for infertility that are discussed in this book. We cannot often definitively establish that a partic-

recipe books', in M. M. Dowd and J. A. Eckerle (eds), *Genre and women's life writing in early modern England*, Aldershot 2007, 49–63 at pp. 50–1.

[59] Ibid. 51.

[60] Elaine Hobby, *The virtue of necessity: English women's writing, 1649–1688*, London 1988, 167.

[61] Field, '"Many hands hands"', 56–7.

[62] Leong 'Collecting knowledge', 91.

[63] Sara Pennell, 'Perfecting practice? Women, manuscript recipes and knowledge in early modern England', in Victoria E. Burke and Jonathan Gibson (eds), *Early modern women's manuscript writing*, Aldershot 2004, 237–58 at p. 242; Leong, 'Collecting knowledge', 94.

ular recipe was ever used. Nonetheless, recipe books can provide some of the best evidence of the practice of popular medicine as in numerous instances recipes were accompanied by marginalia and annotations that attest to their use in a specific situation or that suggest that they were used repeatedly. For example in the book attributed to Johanna Saint John, a recipe was recorded with the title 'To Cause Conception Mrs Patricke Conceived Twice together with it & she advised it to one that had been 9 years married on whom it had the same effect.'[64] More commonly recipes were accompanied with the note *probatum est* (or an abbreviated form of this): 'this is proven'. Others said in English that recipes had been efficacious or were accompanied by initials or small drawings that suggested they were marked out as particularly good. Thus recipe books are essential for proving the place of medical ideas and therapeutics in the practice of popular medicine. It should be emphasised that in comparing recipe collections with medical treatises it is not assumed that medical knowledge adhered to a simplistic top-down model of dissemination. The ideas found in popular and medical works intersected and interacted with, and were influenced by, each other.

Sexual, reproductive and bodily knowledge was not presented and accessed only in medical texts during the early modern period. Erotic literature and pornography provided a wealth of information about sexual desire and pleasure. As both Sarah Toulalan and Julie Peakman have argued there was plenty of material available, ranging from expensive illustrated leather-bound volumes accessible only to the wealthy, to inexpensive single printed sheets and works suitable for rudimentary readers.[65] Readers of this material were consequently drawn from a variety of social classes and economic backgrounds. Erotic texts also covered a variety of themes; many were political and religious satires which used sex as a way of denigrating unorthodox religious views.[66] Others were more sophisticated topographical works that explored the human body and sexuality through the metaphors of exploration and agriculture. Yet others, those most commonly referred to in this book, took the form of a dialogue between an older, sexually experienced, woman and an innocent initiate (like *The dialogues of Luisa Sigea* [1660] by Nicholas Chorier), or described the life of a notorious or newly reformed prostitute (like the anonymously authored *The crafty whore* [1658]). All of these works were intended to make readers think about sex and imagine the sexual body. They did not however exclude medical, and anatomical, information. Both Karen Harvey and Toulalan have demonstrated that erotic literature in the seventeenth and eighteenth-centuries maintained a clear

---

[64] WL, MS 4338, fo. 213v.
[65] Sarah Toulalan, *Imagining sex: pornography and bodies in seventeenth-century England*, Oxford 2007, 48–61; Julie Peakman, *Mighty lewd books: the development of pornography in eighteenth-century England*, Basingstoke 2003, 37.
[66] Toulalan, *Imagining sex*, 38.

focus on conception and generation.[67] This intertwining of the sexual and reproductive bodies is crucial to historicising aphrodisiacs and to demonstrating that across many forms of literary endeavour sex and reproduction were always understood to be intimately connected.

It is worth highlighting that the reception and consumption of erotic literature was not limited to men.[68] Peakman has noted that women in particular owned copies of 'explicit medical books', which could serve as informants on conception as well as on the sexual act, such as Nicholas Venette's *Conjugal love reveal'd* and the anonymously authored *Aristotle's master-piece*.[69] Toulalan has also considered the ways in which the ironic dedications of these works suggested that they were 'educational' and beneficial for women, informing them about the sexual body and sexual acts which would indirectly benefit their husbands.[70] Erotic literature also suggested that women could access sexual knowledge without reading. In the literature itself this was portrayed through the dialogue between a young naïve initiate and an older knowledgeable prostitute. We may imagine that in reality it was more common for women to obtain knowledge from family members, neighbours and midwives.[71] The interaction of women inside the birthing chamber, in particular, was supposed to initiate the new mother into the realm of female reproductive knowledge. In this case, though, the acquisition of such knowledge was restricted to married women. Women, then, were able to disseminate and accumulate knowledge about the sexual body and generation based on reading, experience and tradition.

Because these works were addressed to and were likely read by a mixed audience, it makes them particularly relevant for understanding what women may have been expected to do if they or their husbands became infertile or impotent. The responses shown in such texts was varied – including the use of flagellation and separation – yet they also suggest the importance of food and aphrodisiacs in facilitating pleasurable and fertile sex. In the *Dialogues of Luisa Sigea* a 'sweet smelling ointment' is applied to a young bride and her new husband to encourage their ardour, and throughout the treatise foods such as plum cakes and wine are described as essential for reviving a body exhausted by sex, nourishing it and making it ready for further 'bouts'.[72] Erotic texts, consequently, allow us to glimpse the ways in which men and women read about sexual activity and – most important – generative sexual

---

[67] Karen Harvey, *Reading sex in the eighteenth century: bodies and gender in English erotic culture*, Cambridge 2004, 81–9; Toulalan, *Imagining sex*, 62–91.

[68] Ian Frederick Moulton, *Before pornography: erotic writing in early modern England*, Oxford 2000, 55–64.

[69] Peakman, *Mighty lewd books*, 35–7.

[70] Toulalan, *Imagining sex*, 54–5.

[71] Toulalan shows that erotic texts also suggested that midwives were repositories of sexual knowledge: ibid. 54.

[72] Nicholas Chorier, *The dialogues of Luisa Sigea*, Paris [1660] 1890, 27–30, 51–2, 74–5.

activity in a non-medical setting. These readers, however, unlike those of medical texts, were not necessarily actively mining these works for useful information. Karen Harvey has discussed eighteenth-century readers of erotic literature and argued that they 'neither copied erotic depictions of sex nor internalized statements about bodies'.[73] This was because the information related about sex and the body in these works was representational, 'saturated with beliefs, desires and fears'.[74] Thus, this genre can help to establish how far ideas about aphrodisiacs, impotence and infertility were diffused through society, but cannot establish exactly how far they influenced actual sexual or medical practices.

Alongside erotic literature, a range of non-medical popular literature included references to the use of aphrodisiacs and their relationship to fertility. Taken as a whole these genres thus map the ubiquity of the acceptance of ideas about sexual stimulation. They demonstrate the acceptance, modification or rejection of medical theories by the wider populace, and can show which ideas were popular and so were adopted and perpetuated by medical writers. Medical culture both fed into and drew upon the broader cultural and intellectual milieu of the period. Several medical texts described how diagnostic tests and remedies for infertility were drawn from popular culture. Jakob Rueff wrote in *The expert midwife* that 'some old women ... have their signes by which they observe whether the greater sterility of unfruitfulnesse be in the husband, or in his wife'.[75] Similarly, John Pechey explained that to remedy abortion 'our ordinary Women use frequently Plaintain-seed, which they take in the morning to the quantity of half a drachm with Wine and Water, or in an Egg, or Broath, or by it self, almost every day, all the while they are with Child, and with good success'.[76] Sometimes, these comments were included to disparage the practices of untrained healers. However, in other cases, like Pechey, it is apparent that medical writers and trained medical practitioners were willing to accept medical knowledge and remedies that they viewed as effective from a variety of sources.

One genre in particular that had to find resonance with a broad audience in order to be commercially viable was the ballad. These song sheets, often printed on one side of a piece of paper, were produced in large quantities in the sixteenth and seventeenth centuries, with approximately three to four million broadside ballads printed in the second half of the sixteenth century alone.[77] Ballads were intended predominantly for oral dissemination; engaging with both literate and illiterate audiences alike, they were

---

[73] Harvey, *Reading sex*, 10.
[74] Ibid. 10.
[75] Rueff, *The expert midwife*, 18 (irregular pagination).
[76] John Pechey, *The store-house of physical practice: being a general treatise of the causes and signs of all diseases*, London 1695, 405.
[77] Adam Fox, *Oral and literate culture in England, 1500–1700*, Oxford 1964, 15.

to be sung in ale houses and other public areas. To enhance their appeal to both audiences, ballads were often decorated with woodcut images. These may have acted as mnemonics or as signifiers to those unable to read the actual song/poem, allowing them to understand the underlying theme and content. Ballads covered a range of topics dealing with political, religious and social subject matters.[78] Importantly, as Helen Berry has argued, popular literature and ephemera, including ballads, were also an important means of constructing and transmitting ideas about gender roles and relationships.[79] Katie Barclay agreed that the central place of marriage and gender relationships in people's lives was reflected in the themes of popular ballads that discussed impotence and cuckoldry.[80] It is these ballads that are exploited in this book as they demonstrate that women may have been expected to respond to such misfortunes by feeding sexual stimulants to their lacklustre husbands. Yet ballads do not provide unproblematic access to the thoughts and concerns of early modern men and women. It is difficult to establish the representativeness of their opinions and the reactions and responses of contemporary readers.[81] It is also difficult to assess how many people would have seen or heard any particular ballad as access to them was haphazard; ballads on different themes were sold and sung in different places: those detailing the last laments of criminals were more likely to be found at scaffold scenes while those discussing community and social pleasures were common in ale houses, and ballads were often purchased in a bundle providing the consumer with a lucky-dip of material.[82] Despite these difficulties, the consistency of themes across ballads and the reprinting of many ballads suggest that their content was representative of contemporary mind-sets. Moreover, as they were aimed at a broad audience they do provide important evidence for widespread acceptance of ideas about gender relationships, sexuality and medicine. A key element of the marital relations that these ballads describe is the sexual harmony and satisfaction of spouses. These ballads thus include information on the generative process, including barrenness and aphrodisiacs.

When considering aphrodisiacs, ballads conformed to wider moral ideas and made generation and marriage relations synonymous. They elucidate women's expectations of sexual pleasure and gratification from their husbands. In particular they show that women expected to become mothers

---

[78] For examples and further information see the UCSB English Broadside Ballad Archive: www.ebba.english.ucsb.edu.
[79] Helen Berry, *Gender, society and print culture in late-Stuart England: the cultural world of the Athenian Mercury*, Aldershot 2003, 5.
[80] Barclay, 'And four years space', 27.
[81] Berry, *Gender, society and print*, 5.
[82] Patricia Fumerton, 'Remembering by dismembering: databases, archiving, and the recollection of seventeenth-century broadside ballads', in Patricia Fumerton and Anita Guerrini, *Ballads and broadsides in Britain, 1500–1800*, Farnham 2010, 13–34 at p. 16.

and would feel cheated if their husband's body was not able to fulfil this promise. In the *Sorrowful bride* a young woman is married to a husband with no libido and complains

> And here is a sorrow which trouble me sore;
> As having my Maiden-head now to this day:
> Is this not enough to make me run away?
> *Alas! I am almost a weary of Life,*
> *for to live a Maiden, tho' a Marry'd Wife.*[83]

Ballads like this one emphasised that male impotence was closely related to infertility because it necessarily prevented conception. Ballads also show us that infertility was a cause of distress for men and women: the bride in this case is described as severely depressed, and evoked both sympathy and scorn from others. In *The contented cuckold* a husband who was unable to father a child was mocked: 'all his old Cronies did laugh him to scorn'.[84] In *Fumblers-hall* the wives of insufficient husbands were also portrayed as vulnerable to the 'taunts and jeers of my Neighbours, who call me *Barren-Doe*'.[85] Although both partners appear to suffer scorn and derision in these ballads, it is apparent that infertility and sexual failure were presented as predominantly relating to the male body. There is a sense that women who are partnered with men who cannot satisfy them or make them mothers are to be pitied. Ballads consequently support the argument that men and women would have sought remedies for this and attempted to strengthen or reinvigorate the sexual and reproductive body. In several ballads this indeed was referred to as wives took active steps to improve their husband's virility and potency.

Domestic medicine and medical markets

As the variety of literature demonstrates, for those who were suffering from sexual or reproductive dysfunction there was a plethora of information available on how to understand these problems and treat them. Men and women could seek aphrodisiacs, and other cures for infertility, both within the home and in the medical marketplace. There has been much debate about the role and development of the medical marketplace in early modern England, which emphasises that early modern men and women were active, informed and voracious consumers of medical products and services. Help could be

---

[83] Anon., *The sorrowful bride: or, The London lasses lamentation for her husband's insufficiency*, London c. 1682–94.
[84] Anon., *The contented cuckold: or, The fortunate fumbler*, London, 1686.
[85] Anon., *Fumblers-hall, kept and holden in feeble-court, at the sign of the labour-in-vain, in doe-little-lane*, London? 1675, 7.

sought from friends, family, physicians, surgeons and apothecaries, as well as from irregular and itinerant healers.

Yet, as several historians have argued, most treatment occurred in the home as many remedies were cheaper to make domestically and did not necessarily require high levels of medical knowledge or specialised equipment.[86] Elaine Leong and Sara Pennell have argued that in the face of an increasingly sophisticated medical market place and consumer society, 'kitchen physick' did not become gradually obsolete, but rather 'adapted itself to a more kaleidoscopic range of inputs'.[87] Moreover, as Leong has shown from the medical collection of Elizabeth Freke (1642–1714), 'men and women spent considerable time in collecting the know-how to produce medicaments, and in making up various medicines'.[88] It was not just simples, single medical plants and substances, that were used in the home, but more complex remedies. In wealthier households like Freke's, where equipment could be purchased, the production of medicines included distilling waters and making up large batches that could be stored for later use. Recipes for remedies, once perfected, were shared amongst friends and relatives providing medical help that could supplement or replace the prescriptions of a medical practitioner. Domestic medicine was the preferred option for patients who did not have sufficient funds to seek the help of a physician or to purchase remedies made up by an apothecary. Many of the substances described as aphrodisiacs in early modern England were foodstuffs that could be found in the kitchen garden or hedgerow, like carrots, nettle seed and cress. Although it cannot be established exactly how frequently these substances were consumed for this specific purpose, it should be remembered throughout this book that some aphrodisiacs were easily accessible and were likely consumed within the home to aid conception and rectify infertility.

Even though scholars have perpetuated the belief that women were the main repository of domestic medical knowledge and the main providers of domestic care, Elaine Leong has argued that this obscures the complex collaborative nature of medical care in the home.[89] Men also played vital roles in the provision of domestic care. Lisa Smith has shown that, as well as collecting and testing medical recipes, male householders were involved in

---

[86] Louise Hill Curth, 'The commercialisation of medicine in the popular press: English almanacs, 1640–1700', *Seventeenth Century* xvii (2002), 48–69 at pp. 49, 60; Patrick Wallis, 'Apothecaries and the consumption and retailing of medicines in early modern London', in Louise Hill Curth (ed.), *From physick to pharmacology: five hundred years of British drug retailing*, Aldershot 2006, 13–27 at p. 17; Elaine Leong and Sara Pennell, 'Recipe collections and the currency of medical knowledge in the early modern "Marketplace"', in Jenner and Wallis, *Medicine and the market*, 133–52 at pp. 135–6.

[87] Leong and Pennell, 'Recipe collections', 137.

[88] Elaine Leong, 'Making medicines in the early modern household', *Bulletin of the History of Medicine* lxxxii/1 (2008), 145–68 at p. 146.

[89] Leong, 'Collecting knowledge', 94–6.

making medical decisions: whether or not to call a doctor; seeking medical advice on health and regimen; and nursing.[90] Deborah Harkness has also emphasised that English medical culture during this period expressed its curiosity about the body through therapeutics.[91] This fostered a medical environment which valued subjective bodily experience of illness and treatment: both men and women were 'exhorted to engage in medical therapies after arming themselves with knowledge of the body' and a familiarity with humoural medical concepts.[92] Thus, she argued that in this period men and women were encouraged to understand their bodies and their health, engage in seeking out medical advice, and negotiate their own treatment. It is evident then that medical knowledge about potency, virility and conception was not the domain of one sex and that medical practice was not strictly separated into commercial and domestic, nor into male and female, spheres.

Outside the home men and women seeking medical advice and treatment had recourse to a range of medical practitioners. The development of the complex medical marketplace in urban centres and particularly in London has been the subject of extensive investigation by numerous scholars.[93] It is important to understand that medical help could be sought from a range of practitioners, including university-educated physicians, apothecaries, surgeons, empirics, clergymen, charitable women and a host of others, irregular and itinerant. It has been argued that there was approximately one medical practitioner for every two hundred residents in early modern Norwich.[94] Consequently it is apparent that medical aid, both paid for and provided free, was available to those who sought it at all levels of society and geographical locations. It was not only in London, and other large cities, that medical help was readily available: as Ian Mortimer has shown, many medical practitioners also operated in the hinterlands and rural areas.[95] This, he argued, was increasingly the case after the Civil War so that both rural and urban dwellers had similar access to medical practitioners.[96] This spread of medical practice meant that it was likely that the medical under-

---

[90] Lisa Smith, 'The relative duties of a man: domestic medicine in England and France, ca. 1685–1740', JFH xxxi/3 (2006), 237–56 at pp. 242, 244.

[91] Harkness, 'Nosce te ipsum'.

[92] Ibid. 175.

[93] Wallis, 'Medicines in early modern London'; Roy Porter, *Health for sale: quackery in England, 1660–1850*, Manchester 1989; Margaret Pelling, *Medical conflicts in early modern London: patronage, physicians and irregular practitioners, 1550–1640*, Oxford 2003, and 'Medical practice in early modern England: trade or profession?', in Wilfrid Prest (ed.), *The professions in early modern England*, London 1987, 90–128; Mark S. R. Jenner and Patrick Wallis, 'The medical market place', in Jenner and Wallis, *Medicine and the market*, 1–23; Wear, *Knowledge and practice*, 28–9.

[94] Mary Lindemann, *Medicine and society in early modern Europe*, Cambridge 2010, 240.

[95] Ian Mortimer, '"The rural medical marketplace in southern England, c. 1570–1720', in Jenner and Wallis, *Medicine and the market*, 69–87.

[96] Ibid. 81, 78.

standing perpetuated in printed works predominantly printed and published in London was not restricted to urban communities.

Finally it is worth highlighting that when medical advice was sought from a physician, it was not the physician who provided the requisite medications. Physicians gave their patients prescriptions which were then filled by an apothecary. Throughout the period apothecaries also increasingly acted as general practitioners, both diagnosing and providing drugs to their patients.[97] Apothecaries were consequently key members of the medical marketplace from whom aphrodisiacs could be purchased. The range and volume available and the consumption of drugs all increased across the early modern period, particularly during the seventeenth century with the expansion of the British shipping industry.[98] Many of the new goods imported at this time from the Mediterranean, Virginia and the Indies, including spices, were thought by medical writers to be aphrodisiacs. Valeria Finucci has shown that on the continent Venetian and Genoese merchants were selling ginger, aloes, vanilla and cinnamon which were all thought to provoke venery.[99] This suggests that people were able to purchase aphrodisiacs from marketplaces and apothecaries, a trend which may have been reflected in the English setting. Gideon Harvey's *The family physician* (1678) provides further evidence for the availability of these substances in the English market-place. Harvey warned his readers that apothecaries sold their medicines ignorantly and at inflated prices.[100] He provided his readers with a list of the medicinal ingredients that could be purchased from '*Druggists*' in London and their current costs. This list included several noted sexual stimulants including eryngo, galangal, pepper, aniseeds, caraway seeds, coriander seeds, nettle seeds, rocket seeds, cantharides and stag's penis.[101] Harvey's rebuke of the London apothecaries implies that, although potentially expensive, numerous aphrodisiacs were available for sale in London's medical market.

Alongside those medicines purchased specifically from apothecaries, eighteenth-century sufferers from these distressing problems who had the requisite wealth could purchase medicaments specifically designed to counter them from a range of sellers who promoted their wares in advertisements. Medical practitioners had advertised their services and patent medicines throughout the seventeenth century in printed handbills, one- or two-sided

---

[97] Penelope J. Corfield, 'From poison peddlers to civic worthies: the reputation of the apothecaries in Georgian England', *SHM* xxii/1 (2009), 1–21 at pp. 2–4.

[98] Louise Hill Curth, 'Medical advertising in the popular press: almanacs and the growth of proprietary medicines', in Hill Curth, *From physick to pharmacology*, 29–47 at p. 35; Patrick Wallis, 'Exotic drugs and English medicine: England's drug trade, c. 1550–c. 1800', *SHM* xxv/1 (2012), 20–46 at pp. 20, 25–6.

[99] Finucci, '"There's the rub"', 530.

[100] Gideon Harvey, *The family physician, and the house apothecary*, London 1678, sigs A2v–A3r.

[101] Ibid. 115–28.

sheets detailing their place of work, the diseases that they could cure and any medicines that they had for sale.[102] Although a number of these handbills claimed that the healer whom they were promoting treated barrenness and infertility, and although a few stated that they sold medicines to do this, these seventeenth-century examples rarely discussed these medicines or their effects in detail. In the eighteenth century, however, the advertisements produced for the newspapers contained far greater detail about the drugs and their supposed effects.

Printed newspapers followed in the tradition of manuscript newsletters and started to be continuously printed in English from about 1695, when the lapsing of the Licensing Act ended pre-publication censorship.[103] As with many of the genres used for this study, newspapers strove to achieve a diverse audience of urban and rural, high and low, male and female readers.[104] Again this allows us to glimpse what these eighteenth-century writers and sellers believed that their audience would find interesting and relevant. Advertisements were crucial to these periodicals. They could fill up to four-fifths of the publication and they were considered to be a part of the reading material.[105] As the number of newspapers increased it became apparent to some that advertisements placed in only one newspaper might be missed; in response a series of newspapers like the *Daily Advertiser* appeared that specialised in presenting advertisements.[106] Medical adverts were a central element of many newspapers, including regional ones, because the newspapers acted as agents for the sale of these drugs.[107] Some adverts were thus not solicited or paid for, which casts doubt on their ability to demonstrate the popularity of the product being sold.[108] Nonetheless, Jeremy Black has demonstrated that some advertisements were successful, like the advertisement placed for anti-venereal pills in a 1709 edition of the *Review* which boosted sales of the product.[109] Although it is hard to tell how far these advertisements were 'popular' or effective and even though some medical adverts were not paid for, advertisements still suggest, by their nature, some measure of expected return. In the case of aphrodisiac/infertility medicines there was a great consistency in the language and ideas used to sell these

---

[102] For further information on these collections see Kevin P. Siena, 'The "foul disease" and privacy: the effects of venereal disease and patient demand on the medical marketplace in early modern London', *Bulletin of the History of Medicine* lxxv/2 (2001), 199–224.

[103] Uriel Heyd, *Reading newspapers: press and public in eighteenth-century Britain and America*, Oxford 2012, 1; Jeremy Black, *The English press in the eighteenth century*, London 1987, ch i.

[104] Heyd, *Reading newspapers*, 3.

[105] Ibid. 12; Black, *The English press*, 52.

[106] Heyd, *Reading newspapers*, 56–7.

[107] Black, *The English Press*, 53.

[108] Ibid.

[109] Ibid. 61.

products. This demonstrates that the advertisers had a clear and consistent idea of what they thought would sell their products effectively. Consequently these adverts, and the earlier seventeenth-century handbills, can still be used to gain a sense of how a wide eighteenth-century audience perceived aphrodisiacs and how they expected them to work.

Procuring medicaments in this way may have provided men and women with a way of purchasing a treatment without exposing their condition to a medical practitioner. Several seventeenth-century advertisements had played upon the theme of privacy and secrecy as one of the key attributes of this method of seeking help, particularly for the cure of venereal disease. The authors of such handbills pointed out that those who felt ashamed could merely send a letter outlining their symptoms and have a remedy sent to them.[110] Advertisements by female healers claiming to heal barrenness, and other female disorders, gendered the privacy that they offered, noting that they provided cures for 'Women, who, through Modesty, are unwilling to let a Common Physician know their Distempers'.[111] Some eighteenth-century adverts continued to offer this service: medicines for infertility and impotence could be acquired by letter, and suitable payment, without the necessity of a disorder being exposed to family members, medical practitioners or the wider community. An advert for 'The celebrated purifying medicines', which, as well as curing venereal disease, did 'more towards banishing Impotence, Barrenness … than any other Specific in the whole Materia Medica' appeared in the *Middlesex Journal* in 1771.[112] The author of this long advertisement concluded by reassuring customers that 'Persons in the Country, labouring under any of these Disorders, may have the Medicines sent, with the utmost Secrecy, by writing (Post paid) to any of the Booksellers by whom they are sold.'[113] Although this comment was ostensibly about distance, it would have been clear to readers that using the post provided a secret way of procuring a remedy for impotence and barrenness. Nonetheless, privacy may not always have been an option as many more advertisements concluded with brief notes stating that the medicine could only be purchased at certain locations: the 'Prolifick elixir', for example, was only sold at the Two Blue Posts in Haydon-yard.[114] Secrecy in this case would rely upon the ability to send a servant or household member to the designated shop. Nonetheless, the descriptive nature of these adverts makes them a useful source for considering the continuity of popular ideas about aphrodisiac medicine as well

---

[110] For examples of privacy see BL, 551.a.32[157], [22],[183].
[111] Ibid. [193].
[112] *Middlesex Journal or Chronicle of Liberty*, London, England, Saturday, 24 Aug. 1771, issue 375. See also *London Journal*, London, Saturday, 11 Sept. 1725, issue 320.
[113] *Middlesex Journal*, 24 Aug. 1771.
[114] *Daily Gazetteer*, London, Tuesday, 3 May 1743, issue 2453.

as demonstrating the varied purchasing options available to those seeking treatment for infertility.

The flourishing book trade of the early modern period created an interested and informed populace. Early modern men and women understood the reproductive body and reproductive failure. They engaged with this medical knowledge, actively recording and sharing useful information and seeking out medical help for their ailments. This medical help could be obtained in the home or in a lively and complex medical marketplace that supplied the needs of both the wealthy and the poor. It is thus apparent that the understanding of aphrodisiacs perpetuated in a range of medical and popular literature at this time could, if a person so desired, be translated into the consumption of these substances in order to improve fertility.

2

The Reproductive and the Infertile Body

'I shall proceed to unravel the mystrey [sic] of Generation', promised the anonymous author of *Aristoteles master-piece* in 1684.[1] He, like other medical writers across the early modern period, expected that nearly all men and women wanted to know about sex and reproduction.[2] There were many different models and theories about the process of producing new life, termed 'generation'. Medical treatises debated the relative contributions that men and women made to reproduction, the function and nature of menstrual blood, the form of the womb and the differences between the sexes. General medical treatises and treatises devoted to obstetrics also considered in detail the reasons why generation failed. There is not scope in this book for a comprehensive discussion of how reproduction and the development of the child in the womb were thought to occur in this period. Rather this chapter will consider some of the elements of sexual difference and reproduction that were questioned and debated in early modern England. Having illuminated which elements of the reproductive body were particularly controversial, the chapter will then consider what was believed to cause infertility in women and in men. It will emphasise the stability that existed across the period in the theories of reproduction with regard to the importance of seed, heat and sexual pleasure. Although numerous elements of the reproductive body and process were questioned, the elements that were thought to cause fertility remained relatively consistent. Thus it will be possible to understand how it was that medical writers were able consistently to advocate aphrodisiacs for the treatment of infertility.

Before exploring the medical understanding of the reproductive system, it should be noted that early modern medical discourses were dominated by the ancient concept that the body was made up of four humours (blood, yellow bile, black bile and phlegm) that existed in a delicate balance. Each humour corresponded to an element and to a season. The differing levels of these humours within a person created their individual constitution. The predominance of a particular humour manifested itself in certain physical and mental characteristics; a person who was cold and dry, for example, was characterised by the presence of black bile and could be of a melan-

---

[1] Anon., *Aristoteles master-piece: or, The secrets of generation displayed* London 1684, 4.
[2] Nicholas Venette, *Conjugal love reveal'd: in the nightly pleasures of the marriage bed, and the advantages of that happy state: in an essay concerning humane generation*, London [1696] 1720, sig A3r.

cholic disposition. The various levels of a person's humours also indicated the illnesses that they were likely to suffer from. Maintaining the correct balance of bodily humours ensured health; imbalances caused illness, which was usually treated by purging the body of the offending humour.

Thomas Laqueur has argued that the dominant early modern medical paradigm for explaining the sexed body, the 'one-sex' model, conflated the male and female form into two versions of the same anatomy.[3] This model, he further suggested, was not displaced until the late eighteenth century, when a 'two-sex' model of sexual difference, where male and female bodies were perceived as anatomically different, gained hegemony.[4] Laqueur's groundbreaking theory prompted scholars to investigate in much more detail how sex difference was constructed in the early modern period. While many have accepted the fundamental premise of the two versions of the sexed body in the early modern period, Laqueur's theory has been qualified and adapted. In particular it is clear that the chronology that he suggested for the transition between these two models is flawed.[5] Throughout this book I will engage with Laqueur's theory, demonstrating, like other critiques, that early modern theories about sex and the body were both more complex and more muddled than his chronology allows. Both the one-sex and the two-sex models were discussed and accepted during the period, and both had implications for how aphrodisiacs and their functions were understood. Although many medical writers accepted the fundamental anatomical differences of the male and female bodies, they, and the wider populace, still concurrently accepted that the male and female physiology of sex and sexual desire were similar.

Medical writers following the 'one-sex' model positioned men and women hierarchically along an axis based on heat, with hermaphrodites occupying the central position. They postulated that men's hotter bodies allowed the genitalia to protrude outside of the body, while women's colder, imperfect, bodies were inverted and retained the generative organs inside to preserve their vital heat. The similitude between the male and female organs can be seen in early modern anatomical diagrams of the womb, for example in Helkiah Crooke's expansive treatise *Mikrokosmographia* (1615) and the cheap pocket-sized *Somatographia anthropine* (1616) (*see* Figure 1). These

---

[3] Laqueur, *Making sex*, 25.

[4] Ibid. 5–6.

[5] Michael Stolberg 'A woman down to her bones: the anatomy of sexual difference in the sixteenth and early seventeenth centuries', *Isis* xciv (2003), 274–99 at p. 276, and 'Menstruation and sexual difference in early modern medicine', in Andrew Shail and Gillian Howie (eds), *Menstruation: a cultural history*, Basingstoke 2005, 90–101 at p. 93; Mary Fissell, 'Gender and generation: representing reproduction in early modern England', *Gender and History* vii/3 (1995), 433–56; Harvey, *Reading sex*, 5–7, 78–81. For further critiques of Laqueur see Wendy Churchill, *Female patients in early modern Britain: gender, diagnosis and treatment*, Farnham 2012, 142, 177, and Christina Benninghaus, 'Beyond constructivism? Gender, medicine and the early history of sperm analysis, Germany, 1870–1900, *Gender & History* xxiv/3 (2012), 647–76.

showed the womb arranged to match the situation and appearance of the male organs.[6] Crooke was a physician and anatomist who studied medicine at Leiden and Cambridge. His *Mikrokosmographia* was a compilation of current knowledge intended for use as a teaching aid. The text accompanying this image explained how the inversion of the organs was conceptualised:

> [the] wombe is likened by *Galen* ... to the *scrotum* or cod of a man as if the cod were but a womb turned the inside outward, and hanging forth from the Share-bone ... For if a man doe imagine the cod to be turned and thrust inward, betwixt the bladder and the right gut, then the Testicles which were in it will nowe cleave to it outwardlye on either side, and so that which was before a cod will now bee a perfect Matrixe.[7]

The idea that male and female bodies were essentially the same in structure had consequences for how early modern people understood the boundaries between the sexes. Although people were categorised as essentially either male or female (or hermaphrodite), the presentation of secondary sexual characteristics could vary dramatically according to the heat of the body creating variations in degrees of maleness and femaleness. A particularly warm woman could be very masculine, described as a virago, while cold men were effeminate and weak. As sex was not rigidly predetermined medical writers believed that women could become men if their vital and natural heat was raised to the necessary level. A seventeenth-century edition of Ambrose Paré's surgical treatise included the story of Maria Germane who was believed to be a girl until her fifteenth year, when, '[s]he some-what earnestly pursued hogges given into ... [her] charge to bee kept, who running into the corne, [s]he leaped violently over a ditch, whereby it came to passe that the stayes and foldings being broken, ... [her] hidden members sodainly broke forth'.[8] In this instance the heat accumulated during vigorous exertion was enough to push the generative members out of the body changing the girl's sex to male. Heat not only determined the strength of a person's sexed identity, but also determined the strength of their sexual desire. Cold men and women lacked desire and were often unable to reproduce successfully, while warm bodies had a stronger sex drive and were more procreative. Indeed at least one medical writer included excessive sexual activity as a reason why women became viragos.[9] The heat of the body was related explic-

---

[6] Stolberg has noted that some anatomical images were only loosely related to the accompanying text: 'Menstruation and sexual difference', 93–4.

[7] Crooke, *Mikrokosmographia*, 216.

[8] Paré, *Workes*, 974. See also Sharp, *The midwives book*, 81.

[9] John Pechey, *The compleat midwife's practice enlarged in the most weighty and high concernments of the birth of man*, London 1698, 201. Although he did not describe them as viragos Christopher Wirtzung also noted that hot, barren women were desirous of sex: *The general practise of physicke,* London 1605, 295.

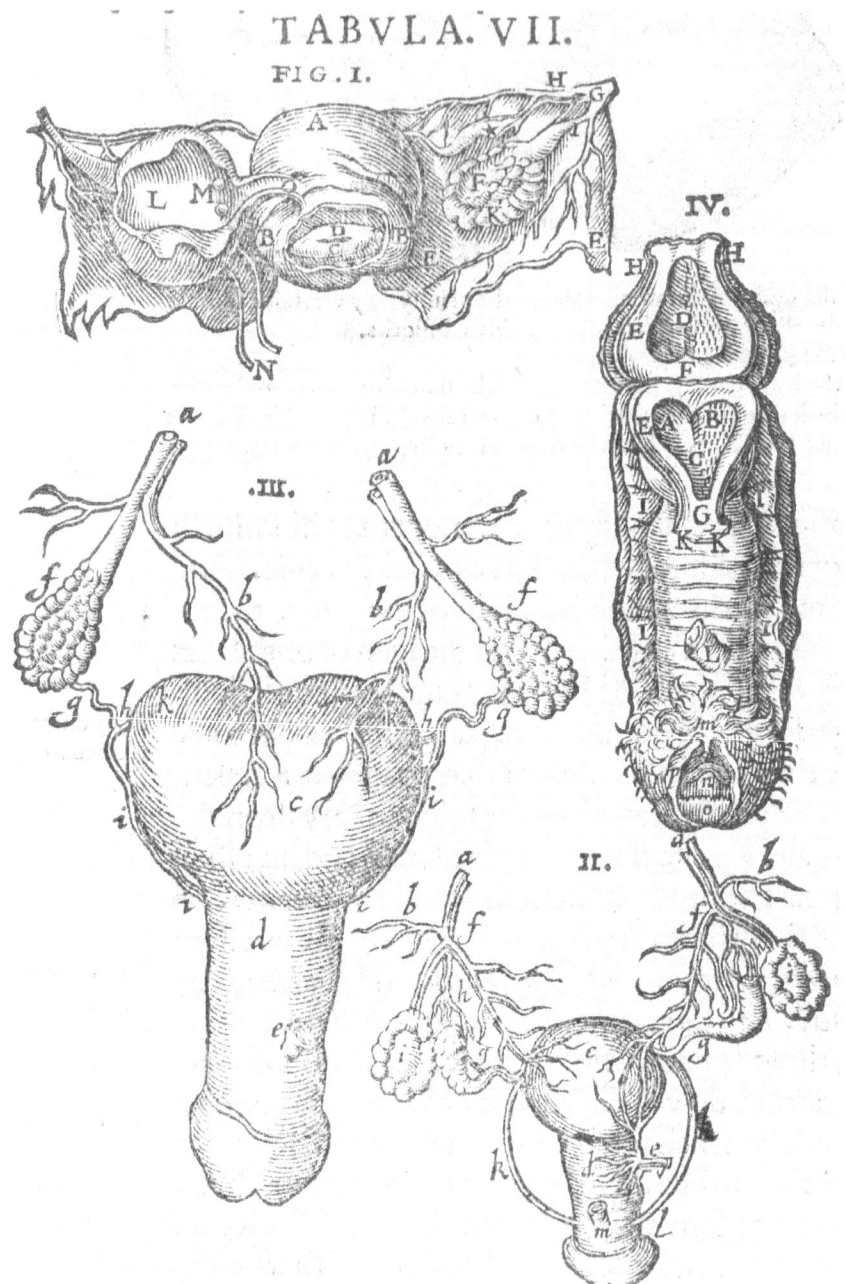

Figure 1. Illustration of a womb and vagina from Helkiah Crooke, *Somatographia anthropine*, London 1616 (The Welcome Library, London)

itly to both gender and sexuality; it categorised people as male or female and allowed them to experience lust and desire.

The idea that men and women's bodies were similar was reflected in the way in which generation and the reproductive organs were described. Women's organs, being imperfect versions of the male anatomy, were generally explained using the available knowledge of the male body, or through comparative descriptions. Even Jane Sharp's *The midwives book* (1671), the first midwifery treatise published by a woman, described women's stones (ovaries) as 'harder and smaller than Mens stones'.[10] Sharp's use of such a linguistic trope perhaps demonstrates the strength of a male-centric model of early modern medicine. However, Wendy Churchill has urged scholars to be cautious in adopting interpretations of such material at face value; she has shown that many early modern writers and healers accepted that women's bodies could exist separately but alongside their male counterparts.[11] Indeed in this case it would seem logical to compare the male and female versions in order fully to understand the feel and size of the organ. Sharp did however assume that a woman's ovaries resembled the male testes and were their equivalent. The use of such tropes did not, as Laqueur's chronology suggested, fall completely out of favour in the late eighteenth century. Writers like Georges Arnaud de Ronsil in his 1763 treatise on disorders of the bladder and urethra, still described the clitoris as 'a small body, whose substance is not unlike that of the *Penis*, nor does it differ in its composition, or figure'.[12] The continued use of such descriptions supported the on-going acceptance of the fundamental similarities of men's and women's bodies.

Laqueur's claim that such a model dominated medical theory until the late eighteenth century was based predominantly upon elite medical treatises and in particular the anatomical images, such as the one above, found in such works. However, considering a broader range of medical and non-medical literature undermines this claim. Stolberg, for example, has shown that from the sixteenth century many medical texts were moving away from the idea of female imperfection towards an understanding of bodily difference and complementarity.[13] Indeed, Helkiah Crooke outlined arguments for both a one-sex and a two-sex model in his work.[14] Even conservative writers, such as Alexander Ross, chaplain to Charles I, argued in 1651 for the presence of two separate anatomies: 'The vessels of generation in the male and female are not the same, as some have thought, supposing they differ onely in scituation [sic], the one being inward, the other outward; which is

---

[10] Sharp, *The midwives book*, 36.

[11] Churchill, *Female patients*, 177.

[12] Georges Arnaud de Ronsil, *Plain and easy instructions on the diseases of the bladder and urethra*, London 1763, 33.

[13] Stolberg 'A woman down to her bones', 274–99 at p. 276, and 'Menstruation and sexual difference', 93.

[14] Crooke, *Mikrokosmographia*, 249–50.

not so, for they differ in figure, number and scituation.'[15] Other writers, like Thomas Bartholin, rather than asserting categorically that there were two different forms, highlighted the ambiguities and confusions inherent in the one-sex model. The 1668 edition of the *Bartholinus anatomy* censured those who expounded Galen's views on the reproductive system for not being clear in their comparisons: was the clitoris or the neck of the womb the penis; and was the womb the female scrotum or part of the glans of the penis?[16] Yet Bartholin himself still employed the descriptive comparisons between the male and female organs in his own work.[17] Accepting the two-sex model, however, did not prevent medical writers and the wider populace from accepting that there were certain necessary elements for fertility that were the same in both male and female bodies.

Before the discovery of the egg and sperm in the 1670s the generative faculty of the body was believed to be seed. Seed was the key component of fertility and sexual pleasure. According to Isbrand van Diemerbroeck's *Anatomy of human bodies*, '*The Seed of man ... is a frothy, white, viscous Liquor, impregnated with a germinating or blossoming spirit, made in the Stones and other Spermatic Vessels of Arterious Blood and Animals Spirits, for the Generation of a like Creature.*'[18] As van Diemerbroeck noted, seed was concocted out of the blood and contained several potent elements necessary for conception. The first of these, he explained, were the salt particles that were separated out from the blood and formed the greatest part of the seed: 'this salt Liquor has the greatest share in the Composition of the Seed, and that its fruitfulness and balsamic Power chiefly proceeds from thence'.[19] Van Diemerbroeck was not alone in arguing that seed was chiefly constituted of salty particles. Jacques Ferrand similarly drew upon the etymology of the words salt and salacious to argue that Venus was born of the salt and of the sea, which explained 'the generative vertue of Salt, which is indeed very great', and that the 'word *Salacitas*, which signifies an earnest desire and appetite to Carnall Copulation, is derived from *Sal*, signifying Salt'.[20] Not all medical writers believed that salty seed was more fertile and excited an itching titillation. As will be demonstrated in chapter 3, several medical writers rejected the idea that seed could be enhanced by consuming brackish and salty foods. Seed also had to contain vital heat in order for conception to occur. Again, van Diemerbroeck explained that '*there is in the Seed of all Creatures, that which*

---

[15] Jonathan Sawday refers to Ross's text as conservative: *The body emblazoned: dissection and the human body in Renaissance culture*, New York–London 1995, 234. See Alexander Ross, *Arcana microcosmi, or, The hid secrets of mans body disclosed*, London 1651, 84.

[16] Bartholin, *Bartholinus anatomy*, 62; Laqueur, *Making sex*, 92.

[17] Bartholin, *Bartholinus anatomy*, 62–3; Laqueur, *Making sex*, 92.

[18] Isbrand van Diemerbroeck, *The anatomy of human bodies*, London 1689, 188.

[19] Ibid. 191.

[20] Jacques Ferrand, *Erotomania: or, A treatise discoursing of the essence, causes, symptoms, prognosticks, and cure of love or erotique melancholy*, Oxford 1640, 246.

renders the Seed fruitful, and is called Heat, *and yet no* Fire'.[21] Helkiah Crooke argued that the man's seed also contained a fragment of the soul which was imparted to the newly-formed foetus in order to create life.[22] Seed was thus a complex liquid that needed to contain the right quantities of heat, salt and spirits in order to be fertile and potent. This understanding of seed was found in a range of literature including a pamphlet satirising the Rump Parliament. *The ladies remonstrance* (1659) lamented the heavy pressure of a dry and withered rump which 'hath neither moisture to *quicken us*, or *heat* to *warm us*; and that we are helpless, and hopeless of any increase or multiplying by the sad distempers of such infirme Members'.[23] The use of generation as an analogy here suggests that the readers of this pamphlet were familiar with the concept of male seed as a hot, moist and potent substance which invigorated new life.

Whether women produced seed or not was widely debated throughout the period. Those who followed the precepts of Galen and Hippocrates advocated that both men and women produced seed, whereas those who adhered to Aristotelian doctrine said that only men produced it. Both of these theories were held concurrently. In Aristotle's view women only contributed menstrual blood to the process of generation, which was formed into a foetus by the active principal of the male seed: as Ross declared in 1651 'there is no active seed in the female for generation, but that she is meerly [sic] passive, in furnishing onely the Matter of Menstruous [sic] blood with the place of conception, is according to *Aristotle* manifest'.[24] The one-seed model was also used for satirical purposes in popular print. The author of the pamphlet *The women's complaint against tobacco* (1675) believed that his readership would accept the idea that women did not contribute active spermatic matter to conception. The author argued that tobacco destroyed men's seed, which was important because 'it is the seed in Man which propagates and begets Children in women'.[25] Here the woman, in line with the one-seed model, was a passive entity carrying a child conceived by the man's seed alone. The existence of women's seed remained contentious in the eighteenth century, with authors continuing confidently to state that women did not produce seed. In 1737 Henry Bracken, a writer on farriery and surgery as well as on midwifery, asserted that 'It would be endless to relate what *Aristotle, Galen*, and other Authors have wrote, with relation to Women's Seed; but their Notions are conjectural, and not founded on Reason. We may be pretty sure

---

[21] Ibid. 194.
[22] Crooke, *Mikrokosmographia*, 259.
[23] Anon., *The ladies remonstrance: or, A declaration of the waiting-gentlewomen, chamber maids, and servant maids*, London 1659, 1–2.
[24] Ross, *Arcana microcosmi*, 36–7 (incorrectly paginated as pp. 60–1).
[25] Anon., *The women's complaint against tobacco: or, An excellent help to multiplication*, London 1675, 3.

that Women have no Semen or Seed, as Men.'[26] Although Bracken rejected Aristotle along with Galen, in rejecting the notion that women had seed he implicitly adopted the Aristotelian one-seed model.

By contrast, proponents of the two-seed model posited that both men and women produced seed which mingled at conception to create the child. This did not negate the role of menstrual blood in the generative process, which continued to provide nutrition to sustain the growing child during gestation. For many medical authors it was clear that both men and women produced seed because God made nothing in vain. Therefore, the presence of testicles in women signified the efficacy of the substance that they produced. Crooke (1615), for example, argued that:

> it is agreed uppon [sic] by all men, as well Physitians as Philosophers, that Nature endevoureth nothing rashly or in vaine. If therefore there bee all Organes for generating, boyling, and deriving or leading seede to the parts of generation in Women as in men, it must needs follow that they also doe generate, boyle and leade downe seed.[27]

Crooke consequently asserted that 'wee have already proved that both the Seedes as well the fathers as the mothers are required in a perfect Generation'.[28] That women sickened if their bodies were not purged of seed through intercourse provided additional evidence that women produced potent seed. It was commonly suggested that the putrefaction of seed retained within the body released damaging noxious vapours into the body that resulted in diseases like the suffocation of the mother and, in virgins, greensickness.[29] This danger was described in both medical and popular literature as a primary reason for a girl to marry.[30] One seventeenth-century ballad advised parents not to withhold their daughters from marriage for fear that they would develop greensickness and seek their own cure through fornication.[31]

Even those who accepted that women produced seed did not always think that it was as potent as men's. Heat was the primary factor that stimulated the concoction of seed and men's greater bodily heat allowed them to do

---

[26] Henry Bracken, *The midwife's companion: or, A treatise of midwifery: wherein the whole art is explained*, London 1737, 15.

[27] Crooke, *Mikrokosmographia*, 283. See also Lemnius, *The secret miracles of nature*, 18.

[28] Crooke, *Mikrokosmographia*, 294.

[29] For example see Culpeper, *Culpeper's directory for midwives* (1662 edn), 108; Sharp, *The midwives book*, 318; Helen King, *The disease of virgins: greensickness, chlorosis and the problems of puberty*, London 2004, 21.

[30] Lævinus Lemnius, *A discourse touching generation*, London 1664, 74; Patricia Crawford, 'Sexual knowledge in England, 1500–1750', in Roy Porter and Mikuláš Teich (eds), *Sexual knowledge, sexual science: the history of attitudes to sexuality*, Cambridge–New York 1994, 82–106 at p. 95.

[31] Anon., *A remedy for the green sickness*, London 1678–80.

this more efficiently. Women were unable to transmute all of their food into blood (hence women were fatty and soft), or to elaborate it further into strong potent seed like their male counterparts. Crooke argued that women 'ingender a more imperfect seede' which was 'moyst, thinne and waterish'.[32] The weakness of women's seed secured the male role in generation; it was only the man's contribution that contained the vital heat required to create a new life. This assertion was vital as the two-seed model raised anxieties that women would be able to conceive on their own. As Ross disdainfully outlined, 'if the females seed were active, shee [sic] may conceive of her selfe without the help of the male, seeing she hath an active and a passive principle, to wit, seed & blood; and where these principles are, there will be action and passion'.[33] The removal of the male body from the process of generation was entirely counter-intuitive, and contradicted the idea that God made nothing in vain.

The Hippocratic model was even more complex. It suggested that both men and women were capable of producing hot and cold seed regardless of the sex of the producer.[34] Warm seed, it was thought, would produce male progeny while cold seed would result in the formation of a female foetus. Although it was not always rejected outright, few medical writers explicitly advocated this model.[35] It was perhaps particularly difficult for authors to assimilate this theory within their broader understandings of the body and reproduction precisely because it did not automatically substantiate existing gender hierarchies by attributing the dominant and active contribution to generation to men. However, heating aphrodisiacs did draw upon the idea that heating the seed of men and women would increase the chances of a male child being conceived.

All versions of the two-seed model argued that both men and women needed to ejaculate, hence to experience orgasm, for conception to occur. Consequently both men and women needed to experience sexual pleasure for intercourse to be fruitful.[36] Conception was most likely if the male and female orgasm was simultaneous, as this would thrust the seeds into the womb at the same moment. In 1636 John Sadler, a physician in Norwich, informed his readers that sometimes conception would not happen because of 'the manner of the act: as when in the emission of the seed, the man is quicke and the woman too slow, whereby there is not a concurse [sic] of both seeds at the same instant, as the rules of conception require'.[37] One response

---

[32] Crooke, *Mikrokosmographia*, 218. See also Sharp, *The midwives book*, 62.
[33] Ross, *Arcana miscrocosmi*, 37.
[34] Laqueur, *Making sex*, 39.
[35] For example see Bartholin, *Bartholinus anatomy*, 55, and van Diemerbroeck, *The anatomy of human bodies*, 205. For more ready acceptance see Crooke, *Mikrokosmosgraphia*, 260.
[36] Laqueur, *Making sex*, 46.
[37] Sadler, *The sick woman's looking glasse*, 118–19.

to this problem was to ensure that the woman was sufficiently warmed and aroused before intercourse, which encouraged the production and ejection of seed.[38] This created a context within which the use of aphrodisiacs was crucial to ensuring that conception occurred.

In the seventeenth century anatomical discoveries were made that radically changed the way in which seed and generation were understood. Both William Harvey in England, and on the continent Neils Steno, began to argue that viviparous animals produced and originated from eggs held in the female testicles.[39] In the 1670s Theodore Keckring then published illustrations of ovarian vesicles, eggs which could be found in both married women and virgins.[40] Similarly, around 1677, Antoni Leeuwenhoek, while conducting observations with a microscope, discovered tiny active particles in semen, spermatozoa, that he termed animalcules.[41] Consequently anatomists, physicians and medical writers began to debate the relative importance of each of these 'new' elements in the process of generation: it was now clear that the 'seed' of each sex was distinct, and so could act in a different manner. However, these innovations were not rapidly absorbed by all English medical writers. While more academic treatises quickly integrated these innovations into the existing medical framework of reproduction, more popular works were slower to change. For some these newly discovered reproductive elements merely provided a new language through which generation could be discussed. Thomas Gibson, in *The anatomy of human bodies epitomized* (1682), cautiously informed his readers that

> We must therefore subscribe to that new but necessary opinion that supposes these little Bladders to contain nothing of Seed, but that they are truly Eggs, analogous to those of Fowl and other Creatures; and that the Testicles (so called) are not truly so, nor have any such office as those of Men, but are indeed an *Ovarium* wherein these Eggs are nourished by the Sanguinary Vessels dispersed through them.[42]

Although Gibson did not include animalcules in his text, by 1698 James Keill could confidently assert that

> There are two principal Opinions about Generation; the first is, that all the Parts of the Body were præexistent [sic] in the Egg of the Female, and that Generation is nothing but the quickening and rendring the *Embrye* fit for the Nourishment and due Augmentation which it ought to have. The other is

---

[38] Ibid. 119.

[39] Matthew Cobb, *The egg and sperm race: the seventeenth century scientists who unravelled the secrets of sex, life and growth*, London 2006, 26–9, 99; William Cowper. *The anatomy of humane bodies with figures*, London 1698, sig. Cr.

[40] Cobb, *Egg and sperm race*, 99.

[41] Ibid. 202–3.

[42] Thomas Gibson, *The anatomy of humane bodies epitomized*, London 1682, 138.

> M. *Leuenhoeck's*, who, by his fine Microscopes, does discover a vast number of Animalcules in the Male Sperm; he says, that they have all the Shapes of our Body, and that they alone are sufficient for Generation.[43]

As this suggests, having accepted the presence of these new reproductive elements, authors debated which was the most significant for successful generation. Initially the egg was considered to be the most important contribution to generation. Leeuwenhoek's discovery of the animalcules allowed medical writers to reassert the prominence of the male contribution, and thus of men themselves, to generation as animalcules demonstrated signs of life, contrary to the static, lifeless, egg. James Blondel (1729) attempted to reconcile this debate, arguing that: 'the Opinions of De Graff and of Leewenhoeck, having on both Sides a great Deal of Truth, and being *partly* grounded upon many undisputable Experiments, and ocular Demonstration[s], 'tis better to reconcile them ... by asserting, that the *Ovum* is the proper *Nidus*, in which the *Animalcule* lodges it self, and by which it is nourished for a Time'.[44] In amalgamating these new ideas Blondel was careful to ensure that the male contribution to reproduction remained the active one, and the most necessary to the process. It is important to emphasise, moreover, that the acceptance of these new reproductive agents did not displace the idea that potent seed was necessary for conception and so seed-stimulating aphrodisiacs were advocated throughout the period.

The other main elements that medical writers claimed were essential for conception were the womb, and menstrual blood. There was some inconsistency in the period with regards to how the womb was perceived. Medical writers argued simultaneously that the womb was merely a passive vessel and that it was an active force in generation, sucking in the seed, and mixing it to form a foetus.[45] There was also some controversy about how many children a woman could carry in her womb at any one time. Outdated modes of thinking perpetuated in some treatises argued that the womb had seven cells or segments that allowed a woman to carry up to seven children, three boys, three girls and one hermaphrodite.[46] Others, like Ambrose Paré's, included the story of a woman who had carried twenty children at once, and had to support the weight of her swollen belly with a scarf.[47] Ballads also tapped into these anxieties: *The lamenting lady* (1620) recounted the story of a woman who vilified a beggar for conceiving twins when she was barren. In return,

---

[43] James Keill, *The anatomy of the humane body abridged*, London 1698, 93–4.
[44] James Augustus Blondel, *The power of the mother's imagination over the foetus examin'd*, London 1729, 109.
[45] Sharp, *The midwives book*, 63; Thomas Raynalde, *The byrth of mankynd, otherwyse named the womans boke*, London [1545] 1552, sig Cxxxviii r; Ross, *Arcana microcosmi*, 88; Crawford, *Blood, bodies and families*, 58.
[46] Sharp, *The midwives book*, 69; Raynalde, *The byrth of mankynd*, fo. Xi r–v.
[47] Paré, *Workes*, 971.

and in response to the beggar's prayers, God made the Lady deliver 'as many children at one time, as daies were in the yeare'; the children 'in bignesse all like new bred mice' died quickly and were buried in one grave.[48] Excessive fertility provoked anxiety because it could result in the birth of numerous children who drained the financial resources of their parents, or, more alarmingly, those of the parish. However, these stories also demonstrated that fertility was still a mysterious phenomenon, and that, as in the case of the lamenting lady, it was malleable by outside influences.

Much more controversial was the form and function of menstrual blood. Patricia Crawford, Bethan Hindson and Sara Read have extensively charted understandings of and attitudes towards menstruation in the sixteenth and seventeenth centuries, and so it is not necessary to explore this in great detail here.[49] Fundamentally there were two schools of thought on menstruation, that which perceived it as a toxic excrement that removed impurities from a woman's body, and that which viewed it as a plethora of healthy pure blood. Both, however, believed that it needed to be purged regularly from the body to maintain health.[50] Crooke explained that Galen, Hippocrates and Aristotle all believed that the menstrual blood was 'of a noxious and hurtfull quality'.[51] Believing that menstrual blood was a putrid and noxious substance meant that taboos developed around having sexual intercourse during menstruation. *Aristoteles master-piece* claimed that conceiving at this time could lead to the birth of monstrous and diseased progeny, and condemned mariners and sailors 'who coming home rashly marry, or run upon their Wives without any due regard to their menstrual courses'.[52]

The more popular theory, though, was that menstrual blood was a plethora shed from women's bodies because of the inefficiency of their digestive process: they could not use all the blood that they 'concocted' from the food that they digested.[53] According to this model menstrual blood was the best and purest blood in the body, providing nourishment for a developing foetus. As Alexander Ross described, 'in sound women, it is as pure as any other blood in the body: For it is appointed by nature for nutriment of the infant, whilst it is in the womb; and after birth it is converted into milk'.[54] However, it still had the potential to be harmful if it remained trapped inside the body. The role of menstrual blood in conception was connected to ideas about seed. Those who believed that women did not produce seed argued that it was

[48] Anon., *The lamenting lady*, London 1620?.
[49] Crawford, *Blood, bodies and families*, and 'Attitudes to menstruation in seventeenth-century England', *P&P* xci/1 (1981), 47–73; Hindson, 'Attitudes towards menstruation', 89–114; Read, *Menstruation and the female*; Shail and Howie, *Menstruation*.
[50] Crawford, *Blood, bodies and families*, 21–2.
[51] Crooke, *Mikrokosmographia*, 288.
[52] Anon., *Aristoteles master-piece* (1684 edn), 49.
[53] Crawford, *Blood, bodies and families*, 22.
[54] Ross, *Arcana microcosmi*, 87.

the woman's menstrual blood that was shaped by the male seed in order to produce the child. Alternatively, those who believed that women produced seed suggested that menstrual blood was only the nutriment supplied for the growth of the foetus. Hindson has shown that by the Elizabethan period few medical men still believed that menstrual blood was shaped by the male seed during conception.[55] The relegation of menstrual blood to a nourishing role, however, did not diminish its importance. Medical writers universally argued that menstrual blood was essential for reproduction, as without it any foetus conceived would die from lack of nourishment.

The language of reproductive failure

As is now apparent, ideas about reproduction were not fixed but changed and shifted across the period. Simultaneously older ideas resurfaced many years after they were originally propounded as later authors drew upon and plagiarised existing works. These changes, and continuities, were reflected in the labels that medical writers used to describe infertility and impotence, including unfruitfulness, sterility, barrenness and imbecility. It is worth briefly charting the changing ways in which the terms 'barrenness' and 'impotence' were used. Initially barrenness and impotence were not strictly defined and were often used interchangeably to refer to a variety of afflictions. During this period, though, a shift occurred in the use of these terms towards more separated and gender-specific terminologies. Yet this shift was neither complete, nor consistent, nor progressive, while the increasingly gender-specific use of these terms by medical writers did not signal a fundamental shift in the aetiologies of infertility. Throughout the period the fundamental causes of infertility in men and women were thought to be the same and remained relatively consistent, although there were of course some causes that were specific to the female – to do with menstrual bleeding – and to the male – to do with the action of the penis.

At the start of the period, a clear mutability existed in the terminology used to describe sexual disorders. Not only could a variety of terms be used interchangeably, but there was little gendered distinction in how they were employed. In *The expert midwife* Jakob Rueff explained, using multiple terms, 'that sterility or barrennesse … is not onely a disability and unaptnesse of bringing forth children in women … but in men also of ingendering and sending forth fruitful seede'.[56] For Rueff, barrenness described a complete inability to conceive children, whether this came from a deficiency in the man's ability to eject seed or in the woman's ability to carry a child to term. Through the work of Rueff and others, such as Philip Barrough, this idea

---

[55] Hindson, 'Attitudes towards menstruation', 92.
[56] Rueff, *The expert midwife*, 11–2 (irregular pagination from p. 192).

continued to carry weight into the seventeenth century.[57] It should be noted, however, that outside of medical literature barrenness incorporated a measure of gender bias. In the Old Testament barrenness was used exclusively to discuss the state of the land or of women, especially with regards to their wombs: in particular, Genesis xi.29 described Abram's wife Sarah as 'barren; [for] she *had* no child'.[58] Some medical writers also drew on this parallel with the land and used agriculture as a metaphor for describing generation: 'The womb is that Field of Nature into which the Seed of man and woman is cast.'[59] This language reflected the desire to view men as the active sex in generation, ploughing the female land and sowing the seeds of new life into it. Some like Thomas Raynalde also described infertility using this metaphor (although he did not use the term barren). He explained that 'yf this sede co[n]ceaved in the bowelles of the earth do not prove or fructyfye, then be thou sure that eyther there is lette in the sower, in the sede, or els in the earth'.[60] Thus, while medically 'barrenness' was used to designate male and female sexual incapacity it also had an implicit cultural understanding, derived from theology, which associated barrenness with women and their reproductive organs.

That gender was not a crucial element in understanding sexual incapacity at the start of the period can be linked to the presence in many texts of the 'one-sex' model, or at least an understanding of the similarities of male and female bodies. Consequently barrenness and impotence could have the same causes and be the same disorders because they occurred in analogous bodies. Although there were gender-specific causes for barrenness and impotence, many were innately based upon humoural principles which affected both men and women. As a result, it was not necessary to understand which gender-specific disorder was preventing a couple from conceiving. Treatment could progress on the basis of general humoural theory using aphrodisiac substances to enhance the heat and fertility of both male and female bodies.

As authors increasingly noted the differences between the male and female generative organs, the connection between barrenness and the womb became more pronounced. Accordingly, a clearer gender distinction appeared in the terminology of reproductive disorders. However, this is not to imply that female 'barrenness' excluded disorders that we would consider as impotence or an inability to have sex, like physical malformations. In the seventeenth century Nicholas Culpeper wrote in his *Directory for midwives* (1676) that 'a

---

[57] Barrough, *The methode of phisicke*, 157.
[58] Robert Carroll and Stephen Prickett (eds), *The Bible; authorized King James version with Apocrypha*, Oxford 1998, 12, 35. 'Fruitful' and 'unfruitful' were also terms used in the Bible.
[59] Sharp, *The midwives book*, 63; Raynalde, *The byrth of mankynd*, sig cxxxviii r.
[60] Raynalde, *The byrth of mankynd*, sig cxxxviii v.

cold and dry Womb is commonly barren'.⁶¹ Similarly, in the *Companion for midwives* (1699), Robert Barret described how "tis a duty Incumbent upon us to advance the fertility of the womb as much as possible, and assist 'em in the removal of the Impediments that block it up, and condemn it to an empty Barrenness'.⁶² Nevertheless the progression towards a gendered language of reproductive failure was not cohesive or straightforward. In her work of 1671, derived from the works of Culpeper and others, Jane Sharp epitomised the continued tendency to discuss both genders concurrently, stating that the testicles of both sexes were used to make the seed fruitful and that if they were out of sorts in either partner 'they must needs be barren and unfruitful'.⁶³ It is possible that because the works addressed here were midwifery texts, which inevitably focused upon the female body and the womb, they present a distorted picture of the medical terminology. As Elaine Hobby noted, these manuals were a part of the general trend of making medical knowledge available in the vernacular and were not always the work of practitioners.⁶⁴ Yet gender-specific terminology was also employed in more general medical texts. In the 1662 edition of *A golden practice of physick* it was stated that barrenness was a disorder found in women 'of an Age to Conceive' who 'hath her Courses naturally, and hath use of a Man, and conceiveth not'.⁶⁵

Barrenness was not the only term to take on gender specific connotations around this time. From the seventeenth century onwards the term 'impotence' was gradually adopted to designate specifically male sexual and reproductive incapacity. Indeed the word impotence was also implicitly gendered as it meant a lack of strength and power, inherently male qualities in this period.⁶⁶ This term however was not used strictly in a modern sense but had a much broader meaning that encompassed erectile dysfunction and a range of other problems that caused infertility. Philip Barrough, who studied at Cambridge and was licensed to practice surgery in 1559, wrote of barrenness in men and women but suggested that 'sluggish impotencie' was more likely to occur in men.⁶⁷ A further example can be found in the *Mercurius compitalitius* of the Swiss physician Theophile Bonet.⁶⁸ The *Mercurius* was

---

61 Nicholas Culpeper, *Culpeper's directory for midwives: or, A guide for women*, London 1676, 22.
62 Robert Barret, *A companion for midwives, child-bearing women, and nurses*, London 1699, 59.
63 Sharp, *The midwives book*, 60.
64 Hobby, *The midwives book*, p. xviii.
65 Felix Platter, *A golden practice of physick*, London 1662, 173. It did go on to acknowledge that barrenness could be caused by a deficiency of male seed.
66 OED, *s.v.* 'Impotent', accessed 13 Sept. 2013.
67 Barrough, *The methode of phisicke*, 142; ODNB, *s.v.* 'Philip Barrow', accessed 3 Nov. 2009.
68 Bonet, *Mercurius compitalitius*.

published in England in 1684, highlighting the slow pace of the transition to a gender-specific understanding of infertility. However, Bonet's text illuminates the specificity with which impotence was attributed to men, and consequently the growing separation of the male generative organs from the female. He related the story of a man who 'came to *Spaw* to get a Remedy for his Impotency'.[69] Furthermore, in his chapter discussing '*Leachery and Impotency*' he wrote almost exclusively of male problems, such as thin seed and premature ejaculation.[70] The increasing use of such language and Bonet's use of particular case studies suggests that it was also becoming more acceptable to label men as sexually and reproductively impaired.

The inclination to discuss and label men's deficiencies separately continued to develop in the eighteenth century. Nicholas Venette's *Conjugal love reveal'd* did not hesitate to use the term in a sex-specific context. He described how one man was cured of his infirmities so that his wife 'never complained of the Impotency of her Husband'.[71] A similarly strong gender distinction in terminology appeared in John Ball's *The female physician* (1770). He wrote 'that many women are unjustly deemed barren, that are not so: for the reason why a woman doth not conceive and bear children, is very often owing to a defect in the man: either from a natural inability or impotency in him, or an acquired one'.[72] In these sources a clear tendency is displayed for attributing impotence to men and barrenness to women.

The development of this gender-specific terminology reflected the increasing scepticism of anatomists and medical writers towards the belief that the female body was merely an inversion of the perfect male. As medical writers increasingly accepted the distinctiveness of the male and female bodies, it became necessary to acknowledge, explain and label male generative disorders separately from barrenness in women. This radically altered the understandings of procreation and reproductive failure by highlighting that reproductive problems were not always the fault of the woman. However, this transition was slow and inconsistent. Throughout the period the understanding of aphrodisiacs continued to draw upon the idea that men's and women's bodies were similar. In most diseases aetiologies were the same for men and women.[73] This was true of infertility where many of the causes, and hence the treatments, were the same in men and women. Despite the similarities in discussions of reproductive failure in men and women, in the rest of this chapter they will be treated in a gender-specific manner for clarity and ease.

---

[69] Ibid. 256, 546.

[70] Ibid. 545–6, 256. The man in the anecdote suffered from both of these deficiencies.

[71] Venette, *Conjugal love reveal'd*, 55.

[72] John Ball, *The female physician: or, Every woman her own doctress*, London 1770, 71. See also Anon., *The ladies physical directory: or, A treatise of all the weaknesses, indispositions, and diseases peculiar to the female sex*, London 1739, 47.

[73] Churchill, *Female patients*, 143.

Understanding infertility

Although there was an upswing in fertility towards the end of the early modern period, medical writers throughout the sixteenth, seventeenth and eighteenth centuries expressed concern that some men and women struggled to conceive. Indeed, François Mauriceau remarked that he 'admire[d] the great passion which many have, who complain of nothing with greater regret than to [be] without Children, especially without Sons'.[74] Medical writers explained, often at length, why men and women became infertile. Principally they argued that reproductive failure was caused by a loss of heat, a deprivation of seed, and a loss of sexual pleasure. These causes remained at the heart of understandings of fertility problems throughout the sixteenth, seventeenth and eighteenth centuries. In turn they were reflected in the various treatments offered by medical writers and practitioners, and were at the root of how aphrodisiacs were understood to be both sexual stimulants and fertility remedies.

Although medical authors outlined numerous natural afflictions that could hinder the fertility of both men and women, all of these disorders were believed to originate from God. God afflicted people with diseases as either a punishment for sin or as a trial of faith.[75] For the godly these tests of faith spurred devotion and prepared the soul for death; for the wicked sickness was a punishment for sin.[76] In most cases God acted through secondary, or natural, methods to create an illness. He also provided medical herbs and knowledge which allowed disorders of the body to be treated. Nevertheless, without God's approval, and often the repentance of the patient, a disorder could not be cured.

This understanding of illness was shared by both Protestants and Catholics, and both doctrinal traditions accepted that fertility was a blessing given by God, and was under his control. Thomas Raynalde's *The byrth of mankind*, a translation of Eucharius Rösslin's midwifery manual, was the first midwifery text printed in English.[77] He stated that 'there is nothynge under heave[n], wych so manifestely & playnely doeth declare and shewe the magnificent mightinesse of the omnipote[n]t lyving god, as doth the perpetual & co[n]tinual generation & co[n]ception of lyving thinges'.[78] It was God's ordinance

---

[74] Hugh Chamberlen, *The diseases of women with child ... written in French by Francis Mauriceau*, London 1672, 6.

[75] David Harley, 'Spiritual physic, providence and English medicine, 1560–1640', in Ole Peter Grell and Andrew Cunningham (eds), *Medicine and the Reformation*, London–New York 1993, 101–17 at p. 101.

[76] Ibid.

[77] *ODNB*, s.v. 'Thomas Raynalde', accessed 14 June 2010. For a comprehensive discussion of Raynalde's treatise see Hobby, *The birth of mankind*.

[78] Raynalde, *The byrth of mankynd*, sigs Cxxxvii v–Cxxxviii r.

to man to populate the earth and increase the numbers of God's holy community. To be barren demonstrated God's displeasure and prevented a person fulfilling their divine duties.[79] Over a century later, in 1671, Jane Sharp also warned her readers of such a misfortune: 'I grant that sometimes *God* is the cause of barrenness, who shuts up the womb, and will not suffer some women to conceive.'[80] Scripture was often used in support of these arguments and in particular the story in Genesis about Rachel who was barren, which led her husband Jacob to prefer her sister Leah.[81] These passages highlight the close relationship between medical understanding and theological influences and shows that medical understandings of barrenness, especially, were shaped by biblical teachings. Fundamentally fertility was given by God, and the restoration of fruitfulness depended primarily upon prayer and the will of God, and only secondarily on medical remedies.

Despite this understanding of God's role in sickness, medical writers tended to remain silent upon this issue. Paul Kocher has observed that Elizabethan works usually only made one or two pious references in the preface and dedicatory epistle and then ignored the supernatural in the main sections on medical practice.[82] This, he argued, was because medical writers realised that ascribing all illness and healing to God marginalised their own role in the practice of medicine.[83] Therefore they emphasised the fact that God acted via natural means to create illness: they focused upon natural causes which were squarely within the remit of physicians.[84] Within this context medical writers were able to explain the virtues of sexual stimulants, as provided by God, and frame their use within the implicit understanding that their effectiveness was governed by God's providence. The idea that treatments would only be effective with God's blessing was particularly invoked by those offering their services via handbills in the seventeenth century: a doctor's wife working in Dean's Court noted that 'as to those whom God hath made *Barren*, none can make them *Fruitful*: But so far as any Obstructions or Impediments may be removed by Art, She will undertake, with God's Blessing to do it'.[85]

In women, medical writers argued that a humoural imbalance of the womb was the primary physical cause of barrenness. This could manifest in several distinct ways. Thomas Raynalde listed the four imbalances that would prevent a woman from conceiving as excessive 'heate of the matrix

---

[79] For a discussion of the religious understandings of infertility see Oren-Magidor, '"Make me a fruitfull vine"'.
[80] Sharp, *The midwives book*, 177.
[81] Ibid.
[82] Paul H. Kocher, *Science and religion in Elizabethan England*, San Marino 1953, p. 264.
[83] Ibid. 266.
[84] Ibid. 269.
[85] BL, 551.a.32 [193].

[womb], over moch coldnes over moche humidite or moystnesse, & over moch dryenesse'.[86] A cold, dense or watery womb could not conceive 'for the powre of the seede is extynguished in it'.[87] The power of seed, especially male seed, came from its heat which gave it the potency to spark a new life. The diminishing of this heat by a cold and moist womb prevented a new life from being created. Raynalde also explained that 'drye matrices, conceave not, for the sede perisheth for lacke of due nutriment and fode'.[88] Here Raynalde referred to a lack of menstrual blood. A dry distemper of the womb also caused the seed to be dissipated or lost. Finally, although a fruitful body required a certain degree of heat to feel desire and to be potent, 'if the womb suffered from extreme and fervent heat … then shall the sede sowen wyther and drye away, & the power of it bee consumed and burnt'.[89] In each of these situations, it was the effects that a distempered womb would have on the seed that hindered conception. A womb that was not correctly balanced was unlikely ever to conceive, or be able to carry a child to term.

The humoural condition of the womb remained a primary feature of infertility discourses throughout the period. In his *Companion for midwives* (1699) Robert Barret expounded that

> *Women* Nevertheless continue Barren; if their Womb be cold, and the Seed be not receiv'd with some wellcome war[m]th, then it slips out again for want of kind Entertainment. Or if the Womb be moist, by reason of the Seed's being choak'd and extinguish'd in the prevailing moisture, which is commonly accompany'd with a cold temperature; or if the Womb be too dry and hot, for then the Seed is burnt up and exhal'd. 'Tis the moderate and temperate constitution that is bless'd with many Children.[90]

Although published at the end of the seventeenth century this description is reminiscent of Raynalde's earlier text, suggesting that Barret had drawn directly upon it or another text that was indebted to Raynalde. An excessively cold and moist womb in particular was described as the most likely cause of barrenness into the later eighteenth century. In 1770 John Ball wrote that, 'the most frequent cause of all, is a cold and moist indisposition of the whole body and womb'.[91] This comment would not have been out of place in any of the texts produced during the period, and emphasises the importance of heat to female sexuality and fertility. The womb existed in a delicate balance. Only when it contained the exact equilibrium of humoural

---

[86] Raynalde, *The byrth of mankynd*, sig. Cxxxix r.
[87] Ibid. sig. Cxxxix r –v.
[88] Ibid. sig. Cxxxix v.
[89] Ibid, sig. Cxl r
[90] Barret, *A companion for midwives*, 62.
[91] Ball, *The female physician*, 71. See also Pechey, *The store-house*, 396.

components did it provide an accommodating environment for the mingling of the seeds and the consequent formation of a foetus.

It was not only the temperament of the womb that could render it barren. Medical writers also explained to their readers that a malformed womb would be unlikely to conceive. For some, including Jakob Rueff, physical malformation was likely to cause untreatable infertility:

> barrennesse may be judged to proceed from the disposition and quality of the generative members: For it commeth to passe, that not a few infirmities and grievances doe happen to them, by reason of which man and wife are not onely made impotent and barren, but are unfit to dwell together ... In which place the strictnesse and narrownesse of the mouth of the Matrix doth very much disprofit and annoy.[92]

Rueff claimed that these physical imperfections, because they caused complete, permanent and un-rectifiable barrenness, necessitated the separation of a husband and wife who had no chance of producing offspring or fulfilling the matrimonial duty of due benevolence; a sentiment that was not reflected in English law. Rueff implied, however, that physical malformation was a less common cause of infertility: it was listed after inconvenient diet, a change of environment, and the drinking of ice water and the use of baths (which cooled the body), all of which affected the humoural constitution of the body and reproductive organs.[93] This may simply have been a reflection of the concerns of medical practitioners who principally discussed disorders for which they could offer treatments.[94] Increasingly in the seventeenth century authors devoted more attention to physical malformation.[95] This may have been a consequence of an increasingly complex knowledge of the physical structure of the womb, acquired through dissection. Many authors also began to explain more clearly that a range of other medical disorders, like tumours and ulceration, could cause physical distortions of the reproductive organs and genitalia that would prevent conception.[96] The treatment of these problems was often described as a two-stage process; first removing the original disease and then progressing to other remedies designed to

---

[92] Rueff, *The expert midwife*, 13 (irregular pagination); Barrough, *The methode of phisicke*, 156–7.

[93] Rueff, *The expert midwife*, 13 (irregular pagination).

[94] Some authors explained that the cure of physical malformations was either impossible or extremely difficult: Platter, *A golden practice of physick*, 176

[95] Culpeper, *Culpeper's directory for midwives* (1662 edn), 1–2. See also Lazarus Riverius, *The practice of physick in seventeen several books*, London 1655, 503; Sharp, *The midwives book*, 165; and James McMath, *The expert mid-wife: a treatise of the diseases of women with child and in child bed*, Edinburgh 1694, 5.

[96] Culpeper, *Culpeper's directory for midwives* (1662 edn), 4–9; Astruc, *A treatise*, 336; Bracken, *The midwife's companion*, 20.

encourage fertility.⁹⁷ In severe cases it was still suggested that the resultant malformation could not be cured and sterility would be permanent.⁹⁸

While the condition of the womb itself was central to infertility, it was also believed that the condition and temperament of a woman's entire body dictated her fertility. Excessive body weight, as Henry Bracken explained, compressed the vagina and so prevented successful intercourse and insemination.⁹⁹ Moreover, weight affected seed production. In overweight people blood was converted into fat rather than into seed, and in lean people it was used up trying to nourish the body.¹⁰⁰ Slender bodies were thought to be unsuitable both for carrying a child to term and for successfully delivery. Moreover, slender women were often categorised as hot and dry and it was thought that they did not produce adequate menstrual blood to nourish a foetus during gestation. Women whose bodies were excessively dry and hot were described as viragoes – dark-haired, lustful, manly and barren. Rueff, for example wrote that these women, 'almost universally, doe want the issuing forth of the Termes at their due seasons, and also the nourishing humours' and consequently are 'not so apt for generation'.¹⁰¹

A lack of menstruation was closely connected to the humoural temper of the body and the womb and was discussed throughout the period. Authors varied in the degree of detail that they provided about this particular problem. Some treatises, like the 1664 edition of Daniel Sennert's *Practical physick*, addressed the issue rather briefly, stating that 'they who want Terms, or have them disorderly, or are sickly, seldom or never conceive with Child'.¹⁰² Other works were more expansive and related a lack of menstrual blood explicitly to the nourishment that the foetus required in order to develop: an edition of Lazarus Riverius' medical treatise explained that a

> defect or badness of the Menstrual Blood, is known, first by the over-great fatness of the whol[e] body, to the nutriment whereof the blood is carried away, and consumed, and is not allowed for the nutriment of the child in the womb. The same is likewise known by great Leanness in the body, and

---

[97] William Salmon, *Systema medicinale, a compleat system of physick theorical [sic] and practical*, London 1686, 241; Pechey, *The store-house*, 396–7.

[98] Salmon, *Systema medicinale*, 240.

[99] Bracken, *The midwife's companion*, 20.

[100] Sarah Toulalan, '"Unfit for generation": body size and reproduction', in Raymond Stephanson and Darren Wagner (eds), *The secrets of generation: reproduction in the long eighteenth century*, Toronto 2014, and 'To[o] much eating stifles the child: fat bodies and reproduction in early modern England, *Historical Research* lxxxvii (2014), 65–93 at p. 78

[101] Rueff, *The expert midwife*, 14.

[102] Daniel Sennert, *Practical physick: the fourth book*, London 1664, 139.

extream slenderness; for when there is not blood enough to nourish the Body, it can hardly superabound to nourish the Conception.[103]

Whether authors fully elaborated on the complexities of this problem or not, it was almost universally acknowledged that menstrual blood was a crucial substance for conception and gestation, and that without it women would be rendered barren.

Eighteenth-century authors continued to outline the importance of menstruation to female fertility. These descriptions continued to focus upon the nutritive role of the menstrual blood. The first treatise written specifically on menstruation, *Emmenologia* (1703), explained that 'the final Cause of the Menses, is agreed by Authors to be, either to render Women more apt for Conception, or to afford Nutriment to the Fœtus'.[104] The author of this treatise, Dr Freind, pointed out that a lack of menstrual blood meant that a woman's reproductive capacities were hindered both because she was not suitable for conception and because she would not be able to support a pregnancy. Like their seventeenth-century counterparts, several eighteenth-century medical writers provided greater details about the bodily disorders that were associated with absent menstruation. Astruc's readers were informed that in women who never menstruated the womb was hard, dense and unsuitable for conception.[105] Henry Bracken, a surgeon and male-midwife, explained that a lack of menstrual bleeding was connected to a disease called the whites, excessive vaginal discharge, which was throughout the period thought to cause barrenness. He explained that this disease caused infertility 'by deriving and exhausting [a] great deal of that Substance, which is re[q]uired for the Nourishment of the *Foetus*: [(] For the *Whites* are a Part of the Blood)'.[106] Bracken was also concerned about excessive menstruation, which he believed caused a moist and slippery temperament in the womb that allowed the seed to slide out after intercourse before, or soon after, conception had occurred.[107] Each of these medical writers believed that menstrual blood was crucial to fertility, and had to manifest itself in regular and adequate menstruation.

Although aphrodisiacs functioned to improve many aspects of the reproductive body, they also provided a direct response to one of the most widely discussed causes of infertility: frigidity, aversion to intercourse and an inability to experience sexual pleasure. This particular problem was intimately related to the cold state of the body. Some medical writers, without

---

[103] Riverius, *The practice of physick* (1655 edn) 505. See also Sennert, *Practical physick*, 134.

[104] John Freind, *Emmonologia: written in Latin by the late learned Dr. John Freind: translated into English by Thomas Dale M.D.*, London [1703] 1729, 4.

[105] Astruc, *A treatise*, 337.

[106] Bracken, *The midwife's companion*, 27–8.

[107] Ibid. 19–20.

considering specifically sexual desire and pleasure, argued that husbands and wives who did not love each other were likely to be barren. For example, Philip Barrough lamented that 'unwilling carnall copulation for the most part is vaine and barren: for love causeth conception, and therefore loving women do conceave often'.[108] Similarly John Sadler in *The sick woman's private looking glass* (1636), which was aimed at a female readership, argued that barrenness was often caused by parents forcing their daughters to marry men whom they did not like, because without love there could be no conception.[109]

That early modern medical discourse described a loss of libido and an inability to experience sexual pleasure as key causes of barrenness demonstrates emphatically that procreation and sexual pleasure were inextricably connected throughout the early modern period. The inability to differentiate between emotional and physical reactions of the generative body to stimuli, such as heat, underscores that for early modern medical writers, practitioners and the wider populace sexual desire and pleasure were paramount in the understanding of generative sex. In the mid-sixteenth century Thomas Raynalde discussed the problem of frigidity in the *Byrth of mankynd*. After explaining a variety of other causes he suggested that some 'woman can not conceave, the cause comming of over moch frigidite and coldenes of the matrixe'.[110] Although Raynalde did not explicitly invoke emotions here his readers would perhaps have already been aware that frigidity manifested as a lack of sexual desire. Seventeenth-century authors were more explicit in connecting the 'psychology' and physiological aspects of this cause of infertility. Popular works like Nicholas Culpeper's *Directory for midwives* informed its audience that the fourth cause of natural barrenness was 'a loss of Carnal Copulation', when 'men and Women come to the School of *Venus* either not at all, or so frigidly, that as good never a whit, as never the better. This is perpetually caused of a cold distemper'.[111] His sentiments were echoed by other medical writers, who, like Culpeper, viewed a loss of desire as a physical state, not a purely emotional disorder.

Many authors were equally emphatic that an inability to feel sexual desire and pleasure was a great impediment to conception. Several of these authors also provided clearer details about why insensibility resulted in infertility. Riverius (1678) explained that

> Among things not Natural, Passions of the mind hold the first rank, and especially hatred between Man and Wife; by means whereof, the Woman being averse from this kind of pleasure, gives not down sufficient quantity of Spirits,

---

[108] Barrough, *The methode of phisicke*, 157. See also Sennert, *Practical physick*, 130.
[109] Sadler, *The sick woman's private looking glasse*, 108–9.
[110] Raynalde, *The byrth of mankynd*, sig. Cxl r.
[111] Nicholas Culpeper, *Culpeper's directory for midwives: or, A guide for women*, London 1651, 87.

wherewith her Genitals ought to swell at the instant of Generation, that her womb skipping as it were for joy, may meet her Husbands Sperm, graciously and freely receive the same, and draw it into its innermost Cavity or Closet, and withall bedew and sprinkle it with her own Sperm, poured forth in that pang of Pleasure, that so by the commixture of both, Conception may arise.[112]

For Riverius a lack of desire prevented the body from producing sufficient quantities of animal and vital spirits that invigorated the woman's seed and encouraged its ejaculation into the womb at the right moment. James McMath's midwifery treatise published one year later similarly informed readers that '*Sterility* happens likewise, from the Womans Disgust, and Satiety of the *Venereal Embrace*; or her dulness, and insensibility therein: Whence the *Orifice* bides shut against the *Yard*.'[113] Here again the womb did not respond to the presence of the man's yard or his seed in the necessary way: it did not draw it in, cherish and nurture it into a foetus.[114] This understanding of barrenness underpinned the discussions of aphrodisiacs as treatments for female infertility in early modern England.

Laqueur has argued that female sexual pleasure became divorced from reproduction in the late eighteenth century.[115] However, medical treatises produced, and reprinted, in the eighteenth century continued to emphasise that a loss of sexual desire resulted in infertility. Throughout the period heat remained a central facet of this understanding of sexual insensibility. The *ladies physical directory* (1739) told its readers that an 'Inappitency to Matrimonial Pleasure', common in women of a cold constitution, 'absolutely prevents Conception'.[116] Similarly, Astruc, who claimed his text was aimed at 'skilful and able judges' of medical theory, wrote that female genitalia which were 'insensible to Love-pleasures' prevented conception and were 'observable in very cold, languid and insensible Women, and th[o]se particularly who hate the Embraces of their Husbands or Gallants'.[117] These statements underscore the continued relationship between sexual pleasure and reproduction, and accentuates that the humoural understanding, which related heat to desire and pleasure, was still fundamental to understanding the fertile and infertile body throughout the eighteenth century.

The final cause of infertility discussed by medical writers was deficient seed production. For those authors who subscribed to the two-seed model of the body, this applied to both sexes. Men and women could fail to produce seed, or could produce seed that was too hot, cold, moist, dry, thick or thin. Moreover, they could produce seed that lacked the elements necessary to

---

[112] Riverius, *The practice of physick* (1678 edn), 503.
[113] McMath, *The expert mid-wife*, 7. See also Sharp, *The midwives book*, 99, 179.
[114] McMath, *The expert mid-wife*, 7.
[115] Laqueur, 'Orgasm', 1.
[116] Anon., *The ladies physical directory*, 51.
[117] Astruc, *A treatise*, pp. v, 336–7.

make it potent, vital heat and spirits. In addition to each of these problems, medical writers also believed that infertility could be caused by the male and female seeds being too constitutionally similar and so not mingling effectively to form a foetus.[118] Although unable to have children as a couple, it was expected that with other more suitable partners these people would have had children. As Riverius explained:

> a certain disproportion or unsutableness [sic] between the Mans Sperm, and the Womans, which makes [sic] they cannot be rightly mingled, nor conspire to the joynt-making up of an Embrion or Rudimental Infant; though there be in the mean while no sensible defect either in the Man or Wife.[119]

In England, barrenness (a lack of children) was not considered to be a suitable reason for separation or divorce, unlike male impotence (which resulted in a lack of sexual intercourse), which was grounds for a separation or in the case of non-consummation an annulment. Yet translations of foreign medical treatises frequently retained discussions of this particular issue. Riverius concluded his own description of this problem by explaining that 'it sometimes happens, that the same man can have a child by another woman, and the same woman by another man; whereas they have lived together in the married estate barren'.[120] An eighteenth-century edition of Nicholas Culpeper's *Directory for midwives* was explicit that 'I know no remedy for it, unless they should part'.[121] Nonetheless, it was also noted in this treatise that this was a rare occurrence 'very seldom found'; rather it was much more common for infertility to be blamed upon a seed deficiency in one partner or another.[122]

It is sometimes difficult in the early literature to identify discussions that specifically reference the problems of deficient female seed. As barrenness designated both male and female infertility it is not always clear which sex's seed is being discussed. However, some writers like Helkiah Crooke were explicit in their descriptions. He argued that the testicles of women functioned to make seed fruitful and thus 'we know assuredly that those women whose testicles are ill disposed are barren and unfruitfull'.[123] Seventeenth-century treatises identified deficient female seed much more readily as a cause of barrenness. An edition of Felix Platter's *A golden practice of physick*, for example, stated that 'it is necessary for Generation that the Womans seed

---

[118] Culpeper, *A directory for midwives* (1651 edn), 83.
[119] Riverius, *The practice of physick* (1678 edn), 504. See also Rueff, *The expert midwife*, 12 (irregular pagination).
[120] Ibid.
[121] Nicholas Culpeper, *A directory for midwives: or, A guide for women*, London 1701, 59.
[122] Ibid.
[123] Crooke, *Mikrokosmographia*, 219.

should be mixed with the mans ... now if the seed be defective, or be in less quantity than is fit, Barrenness is by the womans cause'.[124]

Although the basic aetiology of infertility was believed to be the same in both men's and women's bodies, the inherent differences in the male and female reproductive organs meant that there were some differences in the ways in which men were understood to suffer from reproductive failure. It has often been suggested that because ideals of manhood and patriarchy were reliant upon the assertion of a potent and virile male body, men were rarely held responsible for sexual and reproductive failure.[125] Yet, medical writers clearly accepted that men could be infertile or impotent.[126] To modern readers it would appear that men's reproductive problems were discussed in distinct ways: the inability to have sex – impotence – and the inability to conceive – infertility. This is to a certain extent true – medical writers understood that these two issues were not always synonymous. There was a clear understanding not just of male impotence, but of male infertility. Yet these were considered to be intimately connected disorders. In particular seed was understood to be crucial not just for male fertility, but for sexual desire and the ability to achieve and maintain an erection.

Poor quality or poor quantity seed was also a fundamental aspect of the infertile male body. It was perhaps the primary and most important way in which medical doctrine understood men to be infertile. Throughout the period medical writers lamented that some men produced a paucity of seed because of their poor diet. Seed was concocted out of a man's blood which in turn had been made from his food. Thus without enough or the right sort of food men would become infertile. Jakob Rueff noted that 'sterility and difficulty of ingendring have very great help ... by an unconvenient diet'.[127] Some men, even with the right diet, still did not produce fertile seed. As with women's seed, medical writers like Philip Barrough explained that male seed could be too hot, cold, moist or dry to be potent: infertility 'is of the mans part, when his seede is either hote, & as it were burned, or else cold, thinne, waterie and feeble, as is the seede of old and feeble men: or when it is sent foorth thicker then it ought to be'.[128] Each of these distempers impeded the fertility and potency of the seed meaning that it would not result in a conception. Seed that was too hot consumed and burnt up the potent elements. Conversely, seed that was cold, thin and waterish did not contain enough heat to promote life. Finally seed that was too thick would

---

[124] Platter, *A golden practice of physick*, 175.
[125] Olwen Hufton, *The prospect before her: a history of women in Western Europe, I: 1500–1800*, New York 1995, 177. See also Angus McLaren, *Impotence: a cultural history*, Chicago–London 2007, 75.
[126] Berry and Foyster, 'Childless men', 158–83; Gowing, *Common bodies*, 115.
[127] Rueff, *The expert midwife*, 13 (irregular pagination).
[128] Barrough, *The methode of phisicke*, 157.

not travel to the womb quickly and so would lose its innate heat before it reached its destination.

Concoction was a process that required heat, and, as has already been shown, it was believed that men's innate heat was one of the reasons why men produced better quality seed than women. Cold men, medical doctrine outlined, did not adequately concoct their food and blood into potent seed. Rueff went on to state that 'such men being intemperately cold and moist, cannot send forth seed possessed with a generative vertue'.[129] Seed not possessed of the 'generative vertue' lacked heat and vital spirits. Heat made semen the active element in generation, capable of sparking a new life and imparting a soul. Without this a man's seed was ineffectual. In the seventeenth century Helkiah Crooke discussed the importance of vital spirits, describing how infertility could arise from a deformity in the arteries which supplied the testicles with blood infused with vital spirits that would be concocted into seed.[130] It is unclear whether Crooke viewed the deficient arteries and lack of spirits as two separate causes of infertility. Nonetheless, his statements emphasise the connection between the state of the genitalia and the broader health of the body. The explanations of male seed presented in these early texts demonstrate that male potency primarily relied upon the maintenance of the delicate balance of the constitution and the humours.

The discovery of the animalcules in the 1670s subtly changed the way in which this cause of male infertility was described. Texts such as the *Ladies physical directory* (1739) started to explain that instead of a general problem with the consistency and temperature of the seed, male infertility was directly related to the condition of the animalcules: an 'Effeteness or Infertile Quality of the *Semen*, proceeds from the Want of *Animalcula*, with which, according to the most generally received Opinion, the *Semen* ought to be well stock'd, or from their Languidness.'[131] This description provides a strikingly modern description of infertility caused by a low sperm count or weak spermatozoa that will not impregnate an egg. Still, this passage was included amidst a three-page discussion of the quality of the seed, which relied predominantly on humoural imbalance to explain infertility. In the following sentence the author argued that weakness could be 'for want of the *Semen* being sufficiently Spirituous'.[132] He similarly asserted that '*Semen* is defective in Quality, either when it is of too thick a Consistence, or too thin.'[133] Thus, even though new ideas about the composition of male semen were being incorporated into discussions of infertility, these did not imme-

---

[129] Rueff, *The expert midwife*, 14.
[130] Crooke, *Mikrokosmographia*, 202.
[131] Anon., *The ladies physical directory*, 63.
[132] Ibid.
[133] Ibid. 61.

diately supersede the humoural understanding of potent seed and overall beliefs about the type of seed that would be potent remained consistent.

Poorly concocted seed was, then, unlikely to produce a conception. More than this, thin, weak or cold seed also hindered a man's ability to successfully engage in intercourse. Seed was understood to be both provoked by sexual desire and responsible for creating desire and pleasure in both the man's body and his partner's. A lack of seed or poorly concocted seed was thus intimately connected to a man's libido. Later medical texts, where the term impotence was used with more regularity to describe both sexual and reproductive failure, discuss the potential for men to be ambivalent to sex more than earlier works. This may reflect a tendency on the part of medical writers to assume that male desire for intercourse was the most important factor in a successful conception. Once problems with the male body were recognised as potential reasons for infertility it also had to be acknowledged that men as well as women could suffer from a loss of desire and pleasure. Some categories of sexual stimulants were particularly related to the male body and its potency. These remedies and treatments reflected the fact that medical writers perceived male pleasure as vital to male potency and central to successful copulation.

Throughout the period medical treatises were often unclear about why seed caused pleasure, but they were definitive that this was the case and referred to it itching or stimulating the generative organs as it passed through the seminal vessels. *A golden practice of physick* (1662) elucidated seed's effects upon the penis:

> Venery may be hindered, or weak in both Sexes, if there be either no seed, or at least such as will not provoke the act. For the sharpness of the Seed, causeth the Itch ... and stirs up nature by the spirits, in the Arteries and fils the Spungy Body of the Yard and Glans therewith, so that it is enlarged, swollen, hard, red and hot, and fit for the action.[134]

In this description feeble seed hindered sexual activity for both partners. This probably reflected several ideas: firstly. that if the seed did not titillate the man and cause an erection his partner would be denied any sexual satisfaction; secondly, that in the two-seed model women's seed was also needed to stimulate the female reproductive system; and lastly that male seed was thought to cause intense pleasure for the woman when it touched her womb (this pleasure would be most intense if both seeds were released simultaneously).[135] This 'extraordinary' pleasure, according to Jane Sharp, was a strong indicator of conception.[136] Helkiah Crooke also wrote about

---

[134] Platter, *A golden practice of physick*, 169. See also, Crooke *Mikrokosmographia*, 209, 247.

[135] Laqueur, 'Orgasm', 7; Gowing, *Common bodies*, 119.

[136] Sharp, *The midwives book*, 103. The retention of this idea across the period is unclear;

the stimulating nature of both male and female seed, informing his readers that 'extasie ... is caused by the touch of the seede upon the nervous and quicke sensed parts as it passeth by them'.[137] Again Crooke did not clarify why seed was titillating. Despite the lack of clarity in these texts about the exact process of stimulation, Platter's *Golden practice of physick* was emphatic that potent seed stimulated the male body to engage in intercourse, whereas weak, waterish and crude seed produced 'no pricking, without which there can be no erection'.[138] For these writers, if seed was not potent then it would fail to produce sexual desire, which encouraged a man to engage in sexual activity, and would fail to produce sexual pleasure, which impeded ejaculation and conception. Moreover, the arousing nature of the touch of seed allowed men to maintain an erection, facilitating the stimulation of the female reproductive organs and increasing the likelihood of simultaneous emission of the seeds which would be more likely to result in conception.

Some authors were much more forthcoming about why seed itched and stirred up the reproductive body. For some, like Theophile Bonet, it was the spirituous, acrimonious and salty nature of seed that caused this pleasure.[139] We have already seen that numerous authors believed that it was salt that made seed fertile, which again emphasises the inextricable connection between sexual pleasure and procreation at this time. Without these attributes a man would not feel desire and pleasure in sex, which would in turn hinder his chances of successful ejaculation and conception. However, there was no consensus about what caused seed to be pleasure-inducing. In the early eighteenth century John Marten repeatedly remarked upon the possible effects of seed. In his discussion of impediments to copulation and conception he noted that a defect in the seed could affect desire and pleasure. He wrote that some men were always impotent and unable to enjoy their wives, including those who

> through some defect of *Seed* in the *Stones*, or through the thinness or wateryness of it, have but small inclinations to *Venery*, and when they have, the *Yard* is but faintly erected, and the *Seed* presently or too soon emitted, with very little or no Pleasure to themselves, and as little or less to their Wives.[140]

---

it may be that as interest in the female orgasm declined the pleasurable effects of male seed on the female body were no longer considered. Only a few eighteenth-century treatises rather unclearly mention this issue: Edward Foster, *The principles and practice of midwifery*, London 1781, 28–9; Hendrik van Deventer, *The art of midwifery improv'd: fully and plainly laying down whatever instructions are requisite to make a compleat midwife*, London 1716, 29.

[137] Crooke, *Mikrokosmographia*, 238.
[138] Platter, *A golden practice of physick*, 169.
[139] Bonet, *Mercurius compitalitius*, 694; van Diemerbroeck, *The anatomy of human bodies*, 191.
[140] Marten, *Gonosologium novum*, 21.

As with earlier discussions Marten believed that the thinness and wateriness of seed made it dull and insensible. He did, however, suggest that men suffering from this condition might still be able to engage in some form of intercourse, even if it was short lived. Even more obliquely, an eighteenth-century edition of *Etmullerus abridg'd* simply noted that one of the signs of distempered seed was that 'the venereal Appetite [was] flat'.[141] The author here did not even explicitly state that the seed was stimulating, but only insinuated that potent seed invigorated the desire for sex. Throughout the period then, medical writers willingly accepted that potent seed stimulated and irritated the reproductive organs encouraging sexual activity and making the resultant intercourse more pleasurable. However, they could not necessarily agree on what element of seed actually produced these sensations.

It was not only 'dull' seed that could interfere with male sexual performance. Sharp seed, which was excessively stimulating, and also often thin, as Marten suggested, was thought to cause what is termed today premature ejaculation. This was particularly important in the two-seed model of generation as the emission of the male seed before the woman's meant that they did not meet in womb when both were at the height of their potency. Theophile Bonet described this problem by relating an anecdote about a man who was impotent 'because he let go his Seed at the first touch of the *labia*; but it was watrish and very like whey'.[142] In this situation deficient seed hindered the man's sexual performance. It is unclear whether in such instances premature ejaculation or the quality of the seed was seen as the principal cause of the man's infertility; it is likely that both were considered to be inextricably connected. Bonet explained that such quick ejaculation was a problem because it resulted in the lack of simultaneous emission. He related that 'They whose seed is sharp are excited to *Venus* of their own accord, and quickly emit their Seed, or it runs from them, because of its thinness, without any great sense, and the Member becomes detumescent and languid before … the Woman is ready for expulsion.'[143] Although Bonet related this to thin watery seed, other authors acknowledged that a similar problem could be caused by a weakness of the seminal vessels. In this case, as the author of *The ladies physical directory* observed, the man's seed was potentially potent, but his bodily weakness meant that it was simply shed too soon.[144] The author of this treatise saw this as a particularly debilitating form of impotence, or rather infertility, that 'hinder'd from Fruition, and of Course from propagating their Species, which they can never be able to

---

[141] Michael Ettmüller, *Etmullerus abridg'd: or, A compleat system of the theory and practice of physic*, London 1703, 548.
[142] Bonet, *Mercurius compitalitius*, 256, 546.
[143] Ibid. 545.
[144] Anon., *The ladies physical directory*, 61–2.

do'.¹⁴⁵ However, as Sarah Toulalan has noted, by the end of the eighteenth century at least one author argued that conception was still possible even when the semen had only been deposited within the labia, suggesting that belief in this particular impediment to conception may have weakened by this time.¹⁴⁶

Men, as the hotter sex, were thought to be the most capable in the 'sports of Venus'.¹⁴⁷ Consequently, the suggestion that a man could lose his sexual drive had the potential to damage male patriarchal dominance and physical perfection. Yet medical writers also discussed this possibility without explicitly referencing the man's seed, acknowledging that the cold male body would be frigid, unable to enjoy sex and unable to conceive. Again this was not considered to be a solely emotional problem but was a tangible bodily condition. As with the female body, the understanding that someone could be uninterested in sex and so rendered impotent and infertile encouraged the recommendation of aphrodisiacs as a medicinal substance. It is thus evident that for both sexes throughout the period medical writers did not separate sexual desire and pleasure from reproduction. The physical and emotional states of the generative body remained inextricably connected.

Likewise, medical writers were aware that lust could be tempered and suppressed through the regulation of the six non-naturals (air, food and drink, sleep and waking, movement and rest, retention and evacuation including sexual activity, and the passions of the soul or emotions). In particular it was known that desire could be extinguished by consuming anaphrodisiacs: foods – like water lilies – that cooled the body and provided superfluous moisture. Theophile Bonet opened his discussion of impotence with the observation that camphor cooled the body and when applied to the testicles removed all 'Venereal provocations'.¹⁴⁸ In *Conjugal love reveal'd* Nicholas Venette asserted that 'when Medicines have been inwardly taken, or outwardly applied, to extinguish the flames of Lust, and vanquish the incitements of the Flesh ... the privy Parts are too flaggy and lank, and not able to contribute to Generation'.¹⁴⁹ Despite being induced, and therefore entirely preventable, Venette nevertheless discussed this cause equally with other factors which contributed to impotence. It may be that Venette utilised the idea of an induced state of sexual apathy in order to discuss an innate and natural state, which would perhaps have been embarrassing for men. In adopting this approach he could offer medical advice for this problem

---

[145] Ibid. Premature ejaculation was also associated with gonorrhoea (or gleets) where either disease or an overabundance of seed in the body caused a continual shedding of the sperm.

[146] Toulalan, 'Unfit for generation'.

[147] Nicholas Culpeper, *Pharmacopoeia londinensis: or, The London dispensatory*, London 1653, 31.

[148] Bonet, *Mercurius compitalitius*, 545.

[149] Venette, *Conjugal love reveal'd*, 57.

without explicitly acknowledging that men occasionally suffered a lack of desire. Alongside diet Venette also explained that suffering from a disease could destroy a man's passion because it prevented the body from producing the vital heat and spirits necessary to rouse the generative organs.[150] Other authors agreed with Venette that it was a lack of spirits in the reproductive system that caused men to suffer from diminished libido, but did not tie this only to disease. The *Ladies physical directory* (1739) noted simply that some men wanted 'a *Stimulus* to increase their Amorous Inclinations, rouse their Spirits, and direct or attract them to the proper Parts, so as to enable them to propagate their Species'.[151] Bonet, and the author of the *Directory*, did not make it clear whether this particular problem impeded both sexual ability and fertility, or just fertility alone. Conversely Venette hinted that this problem caused erectile dysfunction, making the male parts 'flaggy and lank'. Again, although this explanation was not always clear, it was apparent to readers of medical treatises that men could be uninterested in sex, through disease, coldness or a lack of vital spirits, and poor seed, which meant either that they did not engage in sexual activity, or that they were inhibited by erectile dysfunction from conceiving.

As with women's bodies, medical writers devoted attention to explaining the physical deformities and malformations of the male reproductive organs that disrupted their ability to have sex and conceive children. These malformations were sometimes discussed in isolation or, particularly in earlier texts, were described alongside problems of the entire body. In the sixteenth century overweight men were believed to be impotent, meaning in some cases that they could not have sex and in others that they were infertile because they could not put themselves into an appropriate position to allow for intercourse (in the approved man on top, face-to-face position) and the quick delivery of the seed to the womb. Both Rueff and Barrough argued that impotence was attributed 'principally to fat men and women, because of the evil proportion, and ill disposition of the generative members, that is to say, in whom the seed is procured and derived from a more remote place'.[152] Obesity elongated the distance seed had to travel to reach the vagina and womb, allowing the seed to cool down. Conversely, a healthy man's seed was cast deep into the womb preventing the loss of vital heat and spirits. Moreover, as in women, body fat was disadvantageous to conception because it removed the majority of nutrition from the blood and therefore prevented the concoction of potent seed.[153]

It was not only obesity that was thought to change the distance that male seed had to travel in order to reach the womb. Medical writers frequently

---

[150] Ibid. 58.
[151] Anon., *The ladies physical directory*, 62.
[152] Rueff, *The expert midwife*, 12; Barrough, *The methode of phisicke*, 157.
[153] Ettmüller, *Etmullerus abridg'd*, 547.

expressed anxiety about the length of the penis and the effects that variations in its form could have on fertility. As Jane Sharp summarised in 1671, 'if the Yard be too long, the spirits in the seed flee away; if it be too short, it cannot carry the Seed home to the place it should do'.[154] A lengthy penis was considered by Sharp to be more of a hindrance; she commented that these men were 'useless for generation'.[155] For Sharp and others, poorly formed genitalia had a negative impact on the seed's humoural balance. Although these men produced potent seed, their bodies did not cherish and deliver this precious substance properly. An abnormally long penis posed further problems to the process of generation according to eighteenth-century authors, including John Marten, who expressed concern that a prodigious member would cause pain and damage the woman during intercourse. Marten explained that 'in the Act of Coition, the *Yard* being forc'd to the very bottom of the *Womb* ... occasioning most cruel Torment, makes the Women cry out, deprives her of her Senses, and quite stupifies her; from which action, if not presently forborn, ensues a great effusion of Blood, Looseness and other Inconveniences scarcely to be remedied'.[156] The damage that Marten described caused two impediments to conception. Firstly it rendered the woman insensible and so prevented her from experiencing pleasure, and potentially releasing her own seed; secondly it caused bleeding and looseness which would have allowed for the man's seed, and her own, to slide out preventing conception from occurring. The length of a man's yard could thus be a cause of infertility, even if it allowed him to engage in sexual activity. Unlike physical malformations in women though, some authors felt that this problem could be aided by the use of cork cushions that artificially reduced the length of the penis.[157]

In addition to the yard's length, medical authors also expressed concern regarding the composition of the generative organs. Every element of the reproductive system had to be in the correct place for it to function properly. In his late seventeenth-century tract *Conjugal love reveal'd*, Nicholas Venette summarised that 'the Yard is also defective when of a little figure, or whe[n] all the little parts it is composed o[f] are not in their right places'.[158] The composition, size and shape of the penis were crucial to successful copulation; there were thus many deformities that could render a man impotent, by either damaging the chances of impregnation or by entirely preventing sexual intercourse. The same concerns were expressed about the testicles. As the producers of seed the testicles were potentially the most important part

---

[154] Sharp, *The midwives book*, 21.
[155] Ibid. 22; Venette, *Conjugal love reveal'd*, 37.
[156] Marten, *Gonosologium novum*, 15.
[157] Ibid. 16; Venette, *Conjugal love reveal'd*, 49.
[158] Venette, *Conjugal love reveal'd*, 40.

of the male generative system. If the testicles did not concoct potent seed then copulation would be entirely fruitless.

Having the wrong number of testicles was frequently discussed by authors in this period and demonstrates their anxieties about the normality of the male generative body. Although medical writers agreed that the wrong number of testicles limited fertility, the appropriate number of testicles was a controversial topic. In an edition of Johan Vesling's *The anatomy of the body of man* (1653) readers were reassured that 'the Divine Creator hath formed two of them, that so the work might be done by the other when the one languisheth, or is deficient'.[159] Nicholas Venette, agreed that one testicle would be sufficient, but added that some men 'have three Testicles, but these have not the Advantages of the former [two]; because instead of being more fertil [sic] by the number of these Parts, they become impotent, the prolifick Vertue being distributed into too many parts to be of any force'.[160] In yet another explanation, the *Bartholinus anatomy*, perhaps uniquely, argued that four testicles were too many and proved barren because they were too small to sufficiently produce seed.[161] The only thing these authors appeared to agree on was that too many testicles caused infertility. Even though the precise number that would result in infertility was contested, medical authors agreed that the fundamental problem was the size of the testicles. Although potentially more numerous, smaller testicles did not contain the necessary twists and turns in the seminary vessels to imbue the seed with spirits, force and potency.[162] The seed that they produced was consequently not strong enough to cause a conception and would not have been titillating enough to cause an erection.

Finally, nearly all medical texts that discussed male virility and fertility described erectile dysfunction as a fundamental barrier to conception, because it barred a man from successfully engaging in intercourse. This problem was discussed as a problem in its own right and in relation to other bodily problems. Throughout the period medical doctrine emphasised the importance of a strong erection to successful generation: Helkiah Crooke wrote in his anatomy that the penis is 'Rigid and straight not onley *ad commodiore[m] coitum*, but also that the passage being open and direct, the seede might

---

[159] Johann Vesling, *The anatomy of the body of man: wherein is exactly described every part thereof in the same manner as it is commonly shewed in publick anatomies ... translated by Nicholas Culpeper*, London [1653] 1677, 23.

[160] Venette, *Conjugal love reveal'd*, 7.

[161] Bartholin, *Bartholinus anatomy*, 55. The relative potency of numerous testicles also appeared in Nicholas Choirer's pornographic work, but did not appear to follow medical thinking on this issue: Toulalan, *Imagining sex*, 14.

[162] Bartholin, *Bartholinus anatomy*, 55. Some authors merely listed that they were usually two in number but that this occasionally differed. See James Drake, *Anthropologia nova: or, A new system of anatomy describing the animal oeconomy ... volume one of two*, London 1717, 117–18.

more freely and directly bee ejaculated or shot foorth.'[163] As Crooke emphasised, the erection of a properly sized penis was vital for transporting seed, and maintaining its vital heat, into the womb. This was reiterated by those writers who argued that the inability to sustain an erection led to infertility. The anonymous author of *The English midwife enlarged* advised readers that 'Another cause of Barrenness by defect of the Yard, is a too much weakness and tenderness thereof, it being not strongly enough erected to inject the Seed into the Womb.'[164] This author did not suggest that problems achieving an erection totally prevented a man from having sex. More important was the fact that even if he managed to penetrate a woman, the ejaculation of the seed was weak and so hindered conception. The focus for these writers was not on sex, but on the fundamental reason for having sex: generation.

Numerous texts explained the internal anatomy of the penis to their readers and described how erectile dysfunction occurred. Earlier in the period these explanations followed the premise that the penis was a hollow space and that an erection was caused by blood, imagination, muscles, pressure, seed and wind inflating the penis.[165] Crooke wrote that 'when as in venerious appetites, the bloud & the spirits do in great quantity assemble themselues out of the veines and arteries, that member is as it were a gutte filled with winde, presently swelling and growing hard'.[166] Consequently, it was believed that men who did not have enough wind in their bodies would be impotent. As more dissections were conducted and medical writers developed new ideas about the internal structure of the penis, they modified these ideas. In the eighteenth century, the *Ladies physical directory* explained that

> THE Nerves supplying those Parts, particularly the Muscles called *Erectores Penis* ... with Animal Spirits, may also chance to be obstructed, either wholly or in Part, so as sometimes to effect those Muscles ... with a *Paralysis*, and either totally or partially disable them from acting or contracting as is requisite for Coition; whence absolute *Impotency* in the first Case, or its next Degree, *Insufficiency* in the last, may ensue.[167]

This text had incorporated some of the new ideas about nervous disorders that were being developed during the early modern period, but also discussed the role of the muscles and animal spirits in facilitating an erection. The continued focus on spirits shows how this author had incorporated these new ideas into the existing framework in order to explain reproductive failure. In this new understanding it was the potential for the nerves and muscles to become obstructed that could completely or partially hinder a man's ability

---

[163] Crooke, *Mikrokosmographia*, 212.
[164] Anon., *The English midwife enlarged*, London 1682, 188.
[165] Eccles, *Obstetrics and gynaecology*, 36.
[166] Crooke, *Mikrokosmographia*, 212.
[167] Anon., *The ladies physical directory*, 62.

to achieve an erection. None the less, what remained constant for these authors was that this would prevent both satisfying sexual activity and the possibility of conception. As Helen Berry and Elizabeth Foyster have also argued medical writers considered impotence to be 'a total incapacity of fruition'.[168]

Overall, early modern medical treatises presented a complex and nuanced understanding of reproductive failure. However, there was a relative consistency across the sixteenth, seventeenth and eighteenth centuries about what was needed for the body to be fertile. The physical form of the body, its ability to produce seed, its vital heat and its ability to experience sexual desire and pleasure were all believed to be vital in ensuring that sex culminated in conception. A deficiency in any one of these elements would prevent potent seed from being produced, from being released at the appropriate moment, from reaching the womb without losing its vital heat or spirits, or would mean that all of this was in vain because the womb failed to cherish and nourish the resulting conception. In particular it was believed that a loss of libido, caused through hatred of one's partner, deficient seed production, or a cold and insensible constitution would destroy fertility. Within this context medical writers, and the wider populace, thus recommended the use of aphrodisiacs to combat infertility in both men and women. Aphrodisiacs increased sexual desire and ensured that men and women engaged in sexual activity. They invigorated the reproductive organs and improved sexual vigour and prowess, which improved the chances of a sexual encounter resulting in conception. The ways in which they were thought to do this, though, closely reflected the ways in which the body was rendered infertile, they supplemented and improved the fundamental elements of fertility including heat, salt and seed. Hence, aphrodisiacs not only encouraged intercourse but made intercourse more fertile.

---

[168] Berry and Foyster, 'Childless men', 169.

3

Provoking Lust and Promoting Conception

'If the barren Woman be naturally cold and insensible of Pleasure during the venereal Action … let the *Remedia Aphrodisiaca* be employed, which are met with almost in all medicinal Books and which should be made hot to warm the Patient.'[1]

In this recommendation, which appeared in his 1743 treatise, Jean Astruc declared that female barrenness should be treated with aphrodisiacs. This typified the way in which early modern medical writers, physicians and the wider populace understood sexual stimulants. In this instance Astruc focused upon how aphrodisiacs that warmed the body and added fuel to the fire of sexual desire could rectify what was recognised as a very common cause of infertility, frigidity. However, his statement could easily have been applied to a range of substances that heated the body, provided nutrition, imbued the body with salt or wind, or that were taken from animals with a lascivious nature, and plants with a phallic appearance. Each of these types of substance were thought to stimulate the sexual organs and to increase the body's desire for sexual intercourse. This was the first way in which aphrodisiacs were considered to be key treatments for infertility; without sexual desire there was no motivation to engage in sexual intercourse and so no chance of reproduction occurring. More than this though, aphrodisiac substances were thought to improve the reproductive potential of the body. When consumed, as will be demonstrated, provokers of lust were thought to cause a range of effects on the reproductive organs and body that increased both sexual pleasure and fertility. Sexual desire and pleasure caused the body to be fruitful, and pleasurable sex was more likely to result in a conception. Medical theory also dictated that procreative sex was more pleasurable. Although not all early modern infertility treatments were aphrodisiacs it is apparent that nearly all aphrodisiacs were thought to be beneficial to the impotent and infertile body.

Medicines at this time were rarely specifics, drugs functioning in just one way or applicable to just one disease. Nevertheless, there were clear taxonomies of remedies that were thought to act in particular ways. William Salmon's early eighteenth-century herbal demonstrated this clearly, explaining the qualities of various drug types such as anodynes (pain relievers), bechicks (abates coughs), cephalicks (medicines appropriate for the head), cardiacks

---

[1] Astruc, A *treatise*, 344–5.

(for the heart) and hystericks (for the womb).[2] Similarly, there were many substances that were well known for their aphrodisiac virtues. Moreover, aphrodisiacs, particularly seed provokers, were a clearly delineated category of medications like those listed above. The intellectual frameworks for understanding aphrodisiacs could be divergent, and sometimes apparently contradictory: medical writers utilised both the humoural model of employing medicines with the contrary quality to the disease for a cure and the idea of sympathy, where substances akin to the disease were used.[3] The unifying feature of these discussions was that, no matter the intellectual model, generally these substances both stimulated lust and improved the fertility of the body. Even though different taxonomies of stimulants are examined here, most aphrodisiacs were thought to combine several virtues and work in numerous ways. Medical authors did not consistently use the designations outlined here to explain the aphrodisiac qualities of a drug. In some cases readers were simply informed that plants and animal substances stimulated lust. The understanding of how aphrodisiacs worked, in all genres, was also not uniform or consistent; substances were disregarded and promoted concurrently. Certain stimulants were rejected towards the end of the period as new ways of thinking about the reproductive organs were gradually adopted. Yet aphrodisiac treatments did not fit neatly within either the one-sex or two-sex models of the body. Even though medical writers increasingly accepted the inherent and fundamental differences between the male and female body, many treatments were thought of as universal – applicable to both the male and the female body. Wendy Churchill has recently argued that even though the drugs and treatments offered to male and female sufferers of many diseases were the same, treatment was always differentiated based upon the physiological differences of the sexed female body.[4] Medical writers did express concern over specifically female physiological functions such as menstruation when discussing barrenness and aphrodisiacs. However, the use of aphrodisiacs to treat infertility does not appear to have been fundamentally 'sexed'. Some drugs were more relevant to either the

---

[2] William Salmon, *Botanologia: the English herbal or history of plants*, London 1710, pp. vi, ix, x.

[3] Even though chemical medicines appeared in the *Pharmacopoeia londinensis* as early as 1618, chemical infertility remedies and aphrodisiacs will not be discussed here because of the difficulties in identifying specifically chemical aphrodisiacs. The attributes of chemical medicines were often based on the original humoural virtues of the substance from which they were taken. Therefore chemical remedies created from known aphrodisiacs may have been recognisable as such. For example it was suggested that chemical physicians recommended the blood of satyrion, which was a renowned aphrodisiac. It is also difficult to ascertain how generally popular chemical medicines were. See Jennifer Evans, 'Procreation, pleasure and provokers of lust in early modern England, 1550–1780', unpubl. PhD diss. Exeter 2010, 218–21, 253–8.

[4] Churchill, *Female patients*, 145–65.

male of female body, but overall most could be given without recourse to specific aspects of either the male or female physiology.[5]

In *Marriage and love in England* Alan Macfarlane suggested that Nicholas Culpeper was more swayed by lust than by a desire for children in his sexual interactions.[6] While for some the pleasure of copulation may have been foremost in their thoughts, this cannot be viewed in isolation. Theologians acknowledged the necessity of sexual pleasure for encouraging men and women to engage in the sexual act, and medical texts explicitly underlined the importance of pleasure in God's work of procreation. For many authors, the role of pleasure was a straightforward motivation to engage in the sinful and shameful act of intercourse. Without this pleasure there would be no generation and the human race would eventually cease to exist.[7] Perhaps the most vociferous pronouncement of this was made by John Marten in the early eighteenth century. He explained that

> God Almighty has ... endued each [sex] with natural Instincts, prompting them to the use thereof with desire, in order to perpetuate the Species, by producing new Creatures to supply the room of those who are gone; without which desire, what rational Creature would have taken delight in so filthy, so contemptible and base thing as *Venery* is? And indeed, had not Nature tack'd a more than ordinary pleasing Sensation and Desire to each Sex, in the Act, by giving those Parts such a quick tender Sense and transporting Titillation, and which with all the artillery of Reason we are not able to controul [sic], (so furious is our passion for the Embrace,) we should have no manner of incitement or inclination to the performing it; and consequently Procreation must soon cease and be at an end.[8]

For Marten and others sexual desire and pleasure were the fundamental motivations to engage in intercourse, without which man would cease to reproduce. In these descriptions sexual desire is never only about sex, but intrinsically about generation. Thus provokers of lust were vital in the maintenance of sexual health. As the posthumous edition of Felix Platter's, *A Golden practice of physick* (1662) emphasised 'the things mentioned to provoke Lust ... are chiefly used for Conception'.[9] Even if an aphrodisiac did not explicitly cause the generative organs to be more fertile, it stimulated the body towards sexual intercourse without which conception could never be achieved. More than this however, early modern men and women understood that sexual stimulants would make them more fertile; pleasure

---

[5] Ibid. 178. Further research would need to be conducted to establish whether medical practitioners did in practice alter their aphrodisiac prescriptions according to the sex of the patient.
[6] Macfarlane, *Marriage and love*, 57.
[7] Crooke, *Mikrokosmographia*, 199.
[8] Marten, *Gonosologium novum*, 1–2.
[9] Platter, *A golden practice of physick*, 176.

and procreation were inextricably linked so that to enhance one was to enhance the other. In this way aphrodisiacs in the early modern period are distinct from modern understandings of sexual stimulants. In modern society lust, and its stimulation, carry connotations of psychological sexual desire, but understandings of sexual pleasure and generative potential in early modern thought flowed into one another and were considered to have the same virtues and qualities. Lust and desire are not universally and consistently understood across temporal boundaries. Although aphrodisiacs could be described in the early modern period using terminology that appears to relate only to lust and the emotions of sexual desire, these terms described physical effects upon the body that related predominantly to the fertility of the generative organs. Knowing that medical writers, and others, rarely distinguished between these effects allows us to understand them and the categories that follow.

Hot foods and heating herbs

One of the most prominent categories of provokers of lust discussed during this period was hot foods. These were foods characterised humourally as hot and that produced a warming sensation when consumed, including meats, herbs and spices. Commonly described heating aphrodisiacs included rocket, mustard, pepper, cinnamon, cress, ginger and warm moist meats. Heat was crucial for desire and so by heating the body these substances increased the desire for and the pleasure experienced in intercourse. This combated the devastating effects of frigidity, which robbed the body of its ability to conceive. Numerous medical writers throughout the sixteenth, seventeenth and eighteenth centuries expounded the virtues of these foods. Jakob Rueff related numerous remedies that were to improve the 'fruitfulnesse' of men and women who were 'hindred very much for want of desire to be acquainted with Venus' which included heating herbs, such as galingale, rocket, pepper, ginger and cinnamon.[10] Rueff did not go into detail about how these foods affected the sensibility or fertility of the reproductive organs, although he did note that these same people might have an 'infirmity of the seeds'.[11] For him it was enough that these substances would encourage men and women to engage in intercourse, thereby overcoming a primary barrier to reproduction. Despite the lack of detail that his treatise provided, the repeated presence of heating foods in his remedies would suggest that the need to heat was a prominent aspect of Rueff's understanding of sexual stimulants.

Even though Rueff's recommendation of aphrodisiacs, on the surface, appeared predominantly to be about ensuring that intercourse occurred, it would have been evident to both him and his readers that hotter genitals

[10] Rueff, *The expert midwife*, 55–61.
[11] Ibid. 55–6.

retained the vital heat of the seed and so increased the fertility of the reproductive body. The ubiquitous nature of these ingredients meant that writers and readers alike understood these plants and spices without the need for detailed explanations of their actions. Rueff, and other authors, including domestic manuscript authors, took it for granted that their readers would understand why particular ingredients had been recommended and how they worked, and so neglected to include this information. Other sixteenth-century authors did not assume that these mechanisms would be implicitly understood and provided clues about why these substances were particularly useful in treating the male genitalia. In one of the first English-language medical treatises, Philip Barrough suggested that the heat of these foods reflected the heat created by friction during intercourse. Barrough argued that one way to improve male sexual desire was to 'let his privie members be continually chafed and rubbed with oyles, ointments and other heating medicines' including pepper and myrrh.[12] He also suggested that 'they which be maried, and cannot use the act of generation, because of the sluggish impotencie and weakenes of their members' should 'use meates that doe heate and engender good humours: as is the fleshe of hennes, capons, partrich, feasauntes, yong doves, birdes of mountains, and specially sparrowes, cockes stones and such like'.[13] It is evident that the heat of these foods and ointments was central to their perceived effects upon lust. Maintaining and increasing the warmth of the body was vital to ensuring conception as well: the penis needed to be warm to ensure that the seed reached the womb in a potent and invigorated state.

In these early examples it is apparent that heat was thought to have an impact on both the male and female reproductive systems. Accordingly it is not surprising to find that many texts suggested that heating foods were aphrodisiacs without explicit reference to the sex of the patient. In the 1658 English edition of Lævinus Lemnius' *Secret miracles of nature* it was noted that those who were infertile should amend their diet to change the 'elementary qualities' of the reproductive organs.[14] Of most benefit, he suggested, were those 'meat[s] as will make them fruitful for propagation; Amongst such things as stir up venery, and breed seed for generation, are all meats of good juice, that nourish well, and make the body lively and full of sap, of which faculty are all hot and moist meats'.[15] Lemnius' loose description suggests that a vast number of hot, and moist, foods were considered to be aphrodisiacs. Moreover, he explicitly regarded these as a means of correcting infertility; they not only stirred up sexual desire but encouraged seed production and made the body lively. Other texts also hinted that these substances

---

[12] Barrough, *The methode of phisicke*, 142.
[13] Ibid. 142 (obscured words filled in from 1590 edition).
[14] Lemnius, *Secret miracles of nature*, 26.
[15] Ibid.

would result in more pleasurable sex by improving the heat of the seed. Many medical writers followed the two-seed model of generation, where both men and women produced seed. Although some readers would have assumed that a male body was being discussed (they were considered to be the norm against which women's bodies were described) unless explicit reference was made to the female body, it is apparent that medical writers did not distinguish between the effects on the male and female body. The popular *Aristoteles master-piece* (1684) wrote that men were stirred up to lust by foods that increased seed production, that were hot and made the body lively and full of sap.[16] The author wrote similarly that women whose cold seed debarred pleasure should eat 'things as are apt to stir up Cholerick, hot humours in the Body, as Anniseeds, or Carraway-seeds'.[17] The touch of seed was thought to be both stimulating and immensely pleasurable. Thus heat not only increased the desire of the body, it also facilitated pleasurable sex. For both of these authors the virtue of heating stimulants was also closely related to the production of seed.

It is perhaps surprising that heating foods were recommended for male bodies when medical authors argued that their bodies were already hotter than women's. Medical writers only rarely warned men that they could overheat their sexual organs by the excessive consumption of aphrodisiacs. Of course one reason for this was that medical writers were addressing these discussions to people experiencing a distemper that caused infertility and so expected their bodies to be cooler. Nonetheless, it is also apparent that heating aphrodisiacs were thought to be particularly relevant to the colder female body. In the seventeenth century several authors discussed heating aphrodisiacs and their ability to increase women's desire and the pleasure that they felt during intercourse. The readers of Nicholas Culpeper's midwifery manual were informed that 'they who have hot wombs, desire Copulation sooner and more vehemently, and are much delighted therwith'.[18] In *The anatomy of humane bodies* (1682) Thomas Gibson further emphasised that there were many arteries in the vagina to increase the flow of blood during sexual congress; these, he stated, 'heating and puffing up the *Vagina* encreaseth the Pleasure'.[19] Thus heating a woman's womb would cause her to experience greater pleasure and make her more likely to conceive. However, this was only when the womb was heated moderately. For authors adhering to the two-seed model, too much heat not only made women sexually voracious, but consumed their seed and made them overly masculine, barren viragoes. Sexuality and fertility required a delicate balance of heat: increasing heat

---

[16] Anon., *Aristoteles master-piece* (1684 edn), 11.
[17] Ibid. 84–5.
[18] Culpeper, *Culpeper's directory for midwives* (1662 edn), 21.
[19] Gibson, *The anatomy of humane bodies*, 153.

improved sexual drive, pleasure and fertility, but too much heat caused barrenness.

Many different foods, herbs and animal secretions that heated the female reproductive system were described as aphrodisiacs. *Aristotle's master-piece* (1694 edition) cautioned, without referencing infertility, that once maids had reached menarche, the onset of menstruation, care would need to be taken as 'if they eat salt sharp things, Spices, &c. whereby the Body becomes still more and more heated, than [sic] the irration and proneness to Venereal Embroces, [sic] is very great, nay, sometimes almost insuparable'.[20] The author did not provide a specific list of substances and thus suggested that all sharp spices could be aphrodisiacs. In this instance the author merely suggested that these foods encouraged girls to engage in sexual activity. Yet in his chapter on sterile women he once again noted that those with obstructions in the vessels had 'small desire to Venery, and the little or no satisfaction received thereby'.[21] This time, where he advocated consuming hot choleric foods, he recommended aphrodisiacs because they made it more likely that a woman would have sex and because they would improve the satisfaction that she felt during intercourse, making her more likely to release her own seed and so making her more fertile.[22]

Unlike those writers who were not always clear about how heat stimulated desire, some writers, who discussed a loss of carnal copulation as a medical problem, provided detailed explanations about the function of heating aphrodisiacs. Even in these chapters, which ostensibly considered libido in isolation from fertility, the discussions were still framed by the understanding that sex was a medical issue because it regulated the body's fluid levels and resulted in reproduction. These writers frequently cross-referenced the information provided in these chapters with their descriptions of barrenness and impotence treatments. Furthermore, in accentuating the multifaceted nature of sexual stimulants these discussions implicitly informed readers that these substances enhanced more than just libido. In the *Mercurius compitalitius* (1684), the Swiss physician Theophile Bonet described several types of sexual stimulants, giving details of how they were thought to work followed by a limited number of examples.[23] He drew upon the understanding that seed was stimulating and fertile because it contained salt particles and heat.[24] Thus he stated that some foods were aphrodisiacs 'by their heat and chiefly by their acrimonious oleous Salt make the Seed more turgid, spirituous and

---

[20] Anon., *Aristotle's master-piece: or, the secrets of generation displayed*, London 1694, 2. The term 'menarche' was not yet in use in this period. Much of this text is based upon Lemnius' *Secret miracles of nature* with some passages reproduced almost verbatim.

[21] Ibid. 79.

[22] Ibid. 80.

[23] Bonet, *Mercurius compitalitius*, 694–5.

[24] van Diemerbroeck, *The anatomy of human bodies*, 191–4.

acrimonious'.[25] Within this category, although it is unclear to what extent the foods were heating as opposed to saline, Bonet listed 'all *aromata*, or spices, and *Balsamick, Sulphareous* [sic] and aromatick things that are of the same nature with these, Cardamoms, Cinnamon, Saffron, Cloves &c. in particular all Pepper'.[26]

Heating aphrodisiacs were also specifically identified in herbals. These texts did not always explain how each plant affected the reproductive organs, or focus on the ways in which they would improve fertility. Yet many authors outlined the humoural nature, hot, cold, dry or moist, of the plants that they discussed. Consequently they informed their readers that plant roots, flowers and herbs that were hot and dry, or hot and moist would stimulate sexual desire and encourage copulation. For example, in *A lytel herball* (1550), attributed to Anthony Askham, it was recorded that savory was hot and dry in the third degree, and that it 'stirreth him tha[t] useth it to lechery, therfore it is forbyden to use it muche in meates'.[27] Likewise the seventeenth-century herbals of John Parkinson and John Gerard both included foods that were described as heating aphrodisiacs. John Parkinson, for example, claimed that mints were heating and 'stirreth up venery or bodily lust' as were cress, mustard seeds and rocket, amongst others.[28] Gerard's *The herball or generall historie of plantes* (1633) listed bastard parsley, wild chervil, saffron, small nettle, the lesser sun flower and burdock in the same manner.[29] In these cases, as with medical texts, it is plausible that the reader was expected to understand the intimate connection between heat and sexual stimulation, and so no further explanation was required. Herbals merely provided a reference for people to find plants that would serve their purpose. This implicit connection demonstrates the strength of the heating paradigm in the application of humoural knowledge to the treatment of sexual dysfunction.

Early modern men and women with a certain level of wealth commonly kept collections of medical remedies in the home, based upon knowledge that they had collected from books and from their own experiments and experiences. These manuscript collections provide a glimpse into men and women's medical understanding and can demonstrate how far ideas about heating aphrodisiacs were accepted by the wider populace. These collections demonstrate that both simple and compound recipes were recorded as able to improve sexual desire. Unlike many of the printed texts, these

---

[25] Bonet, *Mercurius compitalitius*, 694.
[26] Ibid.
[27] Anthony Askham, *A lytel herball of the properties of herbes, newly amended and corrected*, London 1550, sigs jiiv–jiiir.
[28] John Parkinson, *Theatrum botanicum: the theater of plants*, London 1640, 35, 817, 824, 832.
[29] John Gerard, *The herball or generall historie of plantes: gathered by John Gerard of London master in chirurgerie very much enlarged and amended by Thomas Johnson citizen and apothecarye of London*, London 1633, 1023, 1041, 152–4, 207, 707, 751–2, 770, 810–11.

manuscripts explicitly connected heat to improved fertility, not just as a means of ensuring that copulation occurred. The use of simple medicines in these texts may have been because they were easier to use and potentially cheaper. They may also have been used because herbals described an array of plants as sexually stimulating. Rebecca Laroche has shown that a variety of manuscript recipe books include references to material obtained from herbals, including Gerard's *Herball or generall historie of plantes*.[30] In her unpublished recipe book 'A very short and compendious method of physicke and chirurgery' (1642) Jane Jackson recorded that 'to make a woman conceave with childe. Take the roote of Eringium called Sea Holly for it growth by the seaside make it in a sirrup and eate of it in the morning fasting and at 4 of the clocke in the afternoon'.[31] This simple remedy would have been easily prepared in the home and offered a relatively cheap response to infertility.[32] Although Jackson did not claim that eryngo was an aphrodisiac, it was described prevalently throughout medical and herbal literature as a heating sexual stimulant. William Turner's *New herball* described Sea Holly (the common name for eryngo) as having 'the powre to hete', and further explained that 'the use of the roote of thys herbe, to stirre up the lust of the body, and they use to gyve it bothe to men and wymen that are desyres to have chylder' and reiterated a second time that it was used to 'stirre up the pleasure of the body, and to make men and wymen fruytfull'.[33] Likewise, the seventeenth-century translation of Michael Ettmüller's *Etmullerus abridg'd* described how barrenness was to be cured using, amongst other remedies, things that 'gently provoke Venery, *viz*. Satyrion, Eryngo, Rocket and Mustard-seeds'.[34] The appearance of such a well-known aphrodisiac in Jackson's collection implies that it was widely known to improve fertility and to do this through its aphrodisiac qualities.

Although medical authors in the eighteenth century ceased to list numerous heating foods as remedies for infertility, heat was still considered to be titillating and necessary for conception. Jean Astruc's 1743 treatise on diseases in women recommended that aphrodisiac remedies should be 'made hot' to warm a barren patient.[35] For Astruc heat continued to have a direct relationship with the stimulation of desire and pleasure, which was crucial

---

[30] Rebecca Laroche, *Medical authority and Englishwomen's herbal texts*, Aldershot 2009, 12–3

[31] WL, MS 373, fo. 34r; see also MSS 3712, 141; 7391, 68.

[32] John Sadler recommended that barren women should eat candied eryngo root: *The sicke woman's private looking glasse*, 120.

[33] William Turner, *A new herball*, London 1551, 178. For other descriptions of Sea Holly/ Eryngo as an aphrodisiac see Lemnius, *The secret miracles of nature*, 26; Anon., *Aristoteles master-piece* (1684 edn), 12; Thomas Newton, *Approved medicines and coriall receipts*, London 1580, 3; Parkinson, *Theatrum botanicum*, 988; and Salmon, *Botanologia*, 336.

[34] Ettmüller, *Etmullerus abridg'd*, 610.

[35] Astruc, *A treatise*, 344–5.

for ensuring that the vagina and womb were receptive to the penis and male seed.[36] Although the substances themselves were not hot, heat was considered beneficial in the treatment of barrenness. Likewise, in 1770, John Ball recommended that, after purging and correcting medicines, the final step to treating barrenness was that the 'most powerful medicines should be taken, which will warm and invigorate the blood and juices'.[37] The compound remedies that he proposed contained cinnamon, saffron, candied nutmeg, candied ginger and eryngo, as well as a compound made with the tincture of cantharides, itself well-known for its sexually stimulating properties, all of which were known to be heating stimulants.[38] He included alongside these compound remedies a 'prolific elixir' that was described as cordial, stimulating, exciting and enforcing a quick sensation.[39] These authors perceived heat not only as a means of increasing sexual desire, but fundamentally of making the body more fertile.

Eighteenth-century advertisements for patent and ready-made medicines implied that aphrodisiac medicines were useful because they would encourage sexual intercourse, but focused much more on the ways in which heat could improve the fertility of the reproductive organs. These advertisements were designed to appeal to a broad consumer base and so demonstrate that heat was ubiquitously understood outside medical circles as important for improving sexual desire and fertility. Both The *British Journal* and the *Daily Post* advertised the 'Prolifick Elixir', an aphrodisiac remedy sold in numerous newspapers into the 1760s which claimed to be

> A Medicine of inestimable Worth for the Cure of BARRENNESS in Women, and IMBECILITY in Men, and that by promoting the chearful Curricle of the Blood and Juices, raising all the Fluids from their languid depressed State to one more florid and sparkling ... encreasing the animal Spirits, restoring a juvenile Bloom, and evidently replenishing ... the whole Habit with a generous Warmth and balmy Moisture, and thereby envigorating it to such a Degree as not to be imagined ... powerfully strengthens all the animal Faculties and generative Powers in both Sexes.[40]

The name of this remedy clearly advised readers that it was intended to aid fertility: 'prolific', throughout the seventeenth and eighteenth centuries, meant fertile and fertilising.[41] Although a modern reader might not immediately view this as a remedy for male infertility and impotence, the word

---

[36] Ibid.
[37] Ball, *The female physician*, 73.
[38] Ibid. 73–4.
[39] Ibid. 75.
[40] *The British Journal* cx, London, Saturday, 24 Oct. 1724, 4.
[41] *OED*, *s.v.* 'prolific', 10 June 2013.

'imbecility' meant weakness, feebleness, debility and impotence.[42] While many virtues are attributed to this provoking remedy, a clear link is made between endowing the entire body with generous warmth and the invigoration of the generative organs. Evidently the accepted role of heat in sex and conception created a long-lasting medical paradigm in which heating foods and medicines became associated with lust, increased sexual performance and pleasure.

These remedies were rarely sex specific but were used throughout the period to treat both men and women. Very few descriptions in medical texts specified which sex should utilise these remedies and eighteenth-century advertisements nearly always suggested that the remedy worked for both men and women. By not separating the medicines into sex-specific forms it was implied that infertility in men and women was fundamentally the same disorder and could be treated with the same remedy. An early eighteenth-century advertisement for the 'Vivifying Drops for BARRENNESS in Women, and Imbecility in Men' enticed customers with the suggestion of enhanced sexual capabilities and improved chances of conceiving, claiming that the medicine would

> renovate the vital Ferment of the Blood, rectify the languid state of all the Fluids, rouse, fortify, and increase the Spirits, invigorate the Nerves, restore juvenile Warmth and cause a sparkling Gladness and ardent Courage to flow in the Heart, and expand itself through the whole human System ... They potently strengthen and corroborate the parts of Generation, effectually promote Conception, and render both Sexes prolyfick in a wonderful Manner, as Thousands have experienced.[43]

The author of this advertisement strongly suggests that the remedy will function as an aphrodisiac, placing emphasis on the ability of the patient to engage in sexual activities and only noting towards the end that it 'effectually promote[s] Conception'.[44] The intended effects of this treatment further categorise it as a provoker of lust; it increased warmth and the vital spirits and facilitated the production of potent pleasure-inducing seed. The author made no suggestion that these effects would be different in male and female bodies; it simply rendered 'both Sexes prolyfick'. The author presumably believed that readers would accept these unsexed aphrodisiacs and fertility treatments.

---

[42] OED, s.v. 'imbecility', accessed 10 July 2013.
[43] *The Daily Courant* 6309, London, Wednesday 10 Jan. 1722. It also appeared in the *Spectator* cccclix, London, Tuesday 5 Aug. 1712, 1711; the *Whitehall Evening Post* mxxxiii, London, Thursday 22 Apr. 1725, 1718; the *Weekly Journal or Saturday's Post* clvi, Saturday 25 Nov. 1721; the *British Journal* xiv, London, Saturday 22 Dec. 1722, 1722; the *Daily Post* mlxxv, Wednesday 26 May 1725; *Mist's Weekly Journal* vii, London, Saturday 12 June, 1725.
[44] *The Daily Courant*, 10 Jan. 1722.

The advertisement for the 'Confectio Potentissima', which appeared in the *General Advertiser* in 1744, was more assertive in testifying both to the aphrodisiac effects that it induced and to how this in turn improved fertility.[45] The author created a strong impression of the heat of desire that would be fuelled and sustained by taking this medicine. It was still, however, unsexed, described as a remedy for men and women. The corrupted Latin or Italian title suggested that this was a medicine of the highest potency. Readers were advised that the remedy

> enriches the Blood, encreases the Spirits; invigorates the Nerves, and perfectly renovates all the animal Faculties, and generative Powers in both Sexes, to such a Degree as Words can scarcely express; and yet acts not only by a stimulating Quality, or blowing up a Flame, but by adding a true Pabulum Amoris, a kindly Fuel, by which Nature is in a Manner regenerated … impotency and every kind of Weakness, or Imbecillity in the Male Sex, and Barrenness, Weakness, and Inappetency to Conjugal Rites in the Female Sex, are most infallibly and directly cured by it.[46]

It is likely that the authors of these advertisements and the sellers of these medicines adopted this 'unsexed' stance in order to attract as many customers as possible; it was not in their interests to exclude potential purchasers based upon sex or gender. Nevertheless, the number of medicines of this kind offered throughout the eighteenth century suggests that, despite a theoretical move towards the two-sex body, readers of newspapers accepted the fundamental similarities between men's and women's bodies and were willing to purchase medicines designed to work universally. The humoural model of the body constituted it as differentiated by levels of heat, but in the matter of sex and reproduction, all bodies required heat.

One of the most notorious aphrodisiacs of the early modern period was the Spanish fly, or cantharides, mentioned in the recipe above. These small insects were infamous both for their stimulating properties and for the exceptional danger that they posed to the body. Cantharides were ubiquitously understood to heat the body and so were recommended by medical authors in severe cases of sterility. However, it was widely acknowledged that cantharides could over-heat and blister the body, both internally and externally, if not used carefully, and so medical writers repeatedly cautioned against the misuse of this potent remedy. In her seventeenth-century midwifery manual Jane Sharp warned that the consumption of cantharides to stimulate an erection could result in a 'priapisme or continual standing of the Yard', which she considered to be more problematic than if it never stood at all.[47] She continued her caution by highlighting the seriousness of this side effect: 'It

---

[45] *General Advertiser* (1744), London, England, Monday 11 May 1747, issue 3913.
[46] Ibid.
[47] Sharp, *The midwives book*, 30–1.

is not to be imagined what pains some have undergone, who by indiscreet taking of *Cantharides* have fallen into this grievous distemper.'[48] Other treatises also highlighted the range of dangerous side effects that had afflicted those foolish or desperate enough to take this drug. Theophile Bonet recorded that 'I have known several, and among the rest two Noble-men, who used *Cantharides*, the one to gratifie his Whore, the other his new married Wife, but wholly with ill success: For the first fell into a most dangerous pissing of Blood, of which he was Cured with great difficulty: And the other the second day after he was married, died of an Apoplexy.'[49] In the eighteenth century John Quincy claimed that 'They certainly to a strange degree excite Lust, and provoke to Venerey.'[50] Nonetheless, he warned readers of its dangers, telling them of a man 'who by taking a large Dose inwardly, so inflam'd himself, that tho he almost kill'd his Wife ... yet he continu'd even in Distraction with fresh Rage, until he dy'd delirious'.[51] What concerned these authors was that men were apparently willing to risk their health and their lives in order to improve their potency or impress with their virility. However, these discussions also draw attention to the precarious balance of temperature in the sexual body: heat could improve sexual performance and potency, but if too strong could result in blistering, burning and severe bleeding, even death.

Heating aphrodisiacs were evidently popular and widely discussed. One of the reasons why medical writers discussed these substances so extensively was not only that they improved fertility, but that they could help couples to conceive the right child. Heat was the crucial element in producing the perfect male body. The heat of the seed used to create a child determined its sex, as did the side of the womb in which it developed: the right side was warmer and so produced male children.[52] Heating foods were consequently a popular category of aphrodisiacs because they increased the chances of conceiving a male child. The discussion about aphrodisiacs in *The secret miracles of nature* was presented in the chapter on how to conceive a boy or a girl.[53] Similarly in *Aristoteles master-piece*, the advice about curing barrenness occurred in the chapter entitled 'General and particular rules, laid down by learned physicians, how to proceed in getting a Male or Female child.[54] Although the chapter was ostensibly about choosing to conceive a boy or a girl, most of the information provided was directed towards conceiving a

---

[48] Ibid.
[49] Bonet, *Mercurius compitalitius*, 545. See also Marten, *Gonosologium novum*, 44. Apoplexy was a disease akin to a stroke: OED, s.v. 'apoplexy', accessed 8 Aug. 2010.
[50] John Quincy, *Pharmacopœia officinalis & extemporanea: or, A compleat English dispensatory, in four parts ... the fourth edition* London 1726, 174.
[51] Ibid.
[52] Sharp, *The midwives book*, 38, 69; Lemnius, *Secret miracles of nature*, 10.
[53] Lemnius, *Secret miracles of nature*, 25–9.
[54] Anon., *Aristoteles master-piece* (1684 edn), 10.

male child. The author included remedies that would encourage an 'appetite and desire to Copulation'.[55] The author subtly reinforced the necessity of heat for conceiving a boy: he explained that after intercourse the woman should 'gently repose on her right side, with her head lying low, and her body sinking down, that by sleeping in that Posture the cells on the right side of the Matrix may prove the receptacles of the Seed, in which are the greatest store of Generative heat, which is the chief inducement to the procreation of Male Children'.[56] Similarly, in a *Golden practice of physick*, the authors concluded their chapter on barrenness by discussing how 'a Male may be conceived, rather then a Female'.[57] Again the authors reiterated the connection with heat and suggested that this was a common belief: 'some think it may be by their using both a hotter and dryer Diet then ordinary, that Males are gotten, which are of the hottest Nature'.[58] One reason for the popularity of heating aphrodisiacs, then, was that they were thought to improve the chances of the resulting progeny being male.

Nourishing food and seed provokers

Alongside heating foods, medical literature also frequently advocated that barren men and women consume foods that nourished the body and encouraged seed production. The reproductive body concocted seed out of nourishment found in the blood. Helkiah Crooke explained to his readers in 1615 that after the blood had reached every part of the body, superfluous nourishment moved to the testicles and received an irradiation which provided the rudiment of the seed.[59] Therefore, foods that were easily digested, afforded good nourishment and increased the amount of blood in the body were believed to encourage the production of seed, which both generated pleasure and improved the chances of conceiving.[60] Hot foods were considered to be easy to digest and nourishing. The 1595 edition of Thomas Elyot's *The castell of health* explained that hot and moist foods were most like the qualities of the blood and so 'are soone turned into bloud, and therefore much nourisheth the bodie'.[61] Across the period various foodstuffs were recommended

---

[55] Ibid. 10–12.

[56] Ibid. 13.

[57] Platter, *A golden practice of physick*, 177.

[58] Ibid. See also Pechey, *The compleat midwife's practice enlarged*, 275, and Venette, *Conjugal love reveal'd*, 195.

[59] Crooke, *Mikrokosmographia*, 198.

[60] Nicholas Culpeper, *Pharmacopoeia londinensis, or, the London dispensatory*, London 1655, 368.

[61] Thomas Elyot, *The castell of health, corrected and in some places augmented by the first author thereof*, second edn, London 1595, 22.

as provokers of lust because of their ability to nourish the body and breed seed.

In the sixteenth century several authors noted the relationship between nourishing foods and sexual stimulation, without necessarily listing which substances acted in this way. As with heating foods these were often discussed within chapters on barrenness and infertility, highlighting again the context within which they were understood to work. As has already been shown, Philip Barrough suggested that men and women who had suffered a loss of libido should eat meats that 'engender good humours'.[62] He further suggested that these foods would improve the reproductive organs and make them more fertile. In his chapter on sterility he argued that barren women should 'use meates and drinkes easie of digestion, and such as the stomach may well comprehende and consume'.[63] For Barrough, nourishing food was important because it both stimulated the body and improved fertility. Sixteenth-century herbals were clearer about naming those foods that provided nourishment, but only described them as stirring lust, rather than explaining how they aided fertility: William Copland's herbal described how 'Pastinaca' or parsnips did 'engendre thycke blod & much, wherfore it styrreth the luste of the body yf it be much used'.[64] Describing turnip, Thomas Newton similarly explained that the 'seede of the Turnep is very wholsome, and mooveth lust'.[65]

By the seventeenth century medical treatises had also begun explicitly to name the nutritive foods that they regarded as sexual stimulants. In 1640 Jacques Ferrand's French treatise on love/erotic melancholy was published in English as *Erotomania*.[66] Ferrand's tract was intended to prevent his readers from succumbing to erotic melancholy. It thus cautioned that certain foods were liable to stimulate lust and love melancholy: 'Our Patient must abstaine also from all meats that are very Nutritive, Hot, Flatulent, and Melancholy' such as soft eggs, partridges, pigeons, sparrows, quails, hare and especially green geese.[67] Equally, in 1662, *A golden practice of physick* provided a substantial list of foods to correct a 'Want of Copulation'; in particular it was explained that 'we give things that cause seed, and this as we said by its plenty and sharpness stirs up a desire to the Act, and disposeth the members for it. These are such as cause much blood, which is the matter of which seed is made.'[68] The authors also explained that foods that nourished and

---

[62] Barrough, *The methode of phisicke*, 142.
[63] Ibid. 158.
[64] William Copland, *A boke of the properties of herbes*, London 1552, 50.
[65] Newton, *Approoved medicines*, 30.
[66] Ferrand, *Erotomania*. This disease can be thought of as a kind of melancholy or despair caused by erotic passions or unrequited love.
[67] Ibid. 247. A green goose was a very young goose usually killed when less than four months old: OED, s.v. 'Green Goose', accessed 19 Aug. 2013.
[68] Platter, *A golden practice of physick*, 170.

were 'white and full of marrow' provoked lust, such as the brains, stones and flesh of craw-fish, crabs, lobsters, oysters, cuttle-fish, polypus, cocks, quails, sparrows and foxes, as well as, milk, eggs, chestnuts, parsnips, almonds, pine nuts, pistachios, artichokes rapes, beans, peas rice and barley.[69] As can be seen, a large number of substances were thought to be nourishing aphrodisiacs. One clearly defined group of foods in these lists is birds and game which, it would seem, was particularly associated with good nutrition and the production of seed.

These foods were also described as stimulating in non-medical texts. In the 1764 version of *Harris's list of Covent Garden ladies*, the prostitute Miss Bland was noted for her use of aphrodisiacs including oysters, crabs, veal and eggs.[70] The substances that she was described as using appeared in medical treatises as nourishing stimulants. Their appearance in this text suggests, not only that these substances retained their reputation throughout the period, but that they were thought to be extremely potent, causing the prostitute to become savage and wild in her trade. The author of this advertisement was not promoting the use of these substances to help conception. Rather, he focused upon their ability to titillate the generative system and encourage intercourse. This may have been seen as an illicit use of these substances, but it demonstrates that substances thought to improve generative potential could not be separated from those that caused pleasure.

In addition to describing nourishing foods medical writers also wrote about seed provokers. The use of this label may just have been to make it clear to readers what these substances were intended to do. However, it is evident that some foods were not thought to provide nutrition but to encourage the reproductive organs to concoct seed from blood already in the body. Philip Barrough, in addition to his other recommendations, argued that 'it is convenient that you give unto such [people] as desire to get children, some accustomed and pleasant thing to eat or drink before meate, which be most apt to provoke carnall lust, & to ingender seede'.[71] Barrough's description typifies the way in which medical writers at this time could not separate the idea that seed would cause sexual desire and so encourage men and women to have sex, and the idea that potent seed was the primary element of conception. Readers of this text would implicitly have accepted that these aphrodisiacs would both encourage sexual activity and make sex more fertile. *A golden practice of physick*, after describing nutritious aphrodisiacs, added a separate group of seed-provoking foods which included onions, leeks, mushrooms, rocket, coleworts and asparagus.[72] However, the authors noted that these foods often stimulated sexual desire because they were dressed with

---

[69] Ibid.
[70] Rubenhold, *The harlot's handbook*, 155–6.
[71] Barrough, *The methode of phisicke*, 158.
[72] Platter, *A golden practice of physick*, 170.

pepper 'and we suppose that when such things are so eaten it comes rather from the Sawce than the Meat'.[73] This lack of precision in specifying exactly how aphrodisiacs worked was not unique to this text, nor to the seventeenth century. The multifarious nature of sexual stimulants is apparent across the period, especially in the instance of seed production.

In the mid-seventeenth century, Alessandro Massaria, a plague specialist and professor of medicine at Padua, appears to have reserved the highest esteem for seed provokers, recommending their use more than any other stimulant.[74] This is particularly interesting as his text was aimed at a female audience and predominantly discussed women's bodies, which suggests that women had the potential to be titillated by potent seed. (Alternatively he may have expected his readers to employ these foods to treat a deficient husband.)[75] Massaria catalogued a number of substances that 'increase Seed, and incite and stir up Venery', such as 'Eggs, Milk, Rice boyled in milk, Sparrows brains, flesh and bones of all; The stones and Pissels [animal genitalia] of Bulls, Cocks, Bucks, Rams, and Bores.'[76] He then added to the list a number of roots including 'Oynions stewed, Garlick, Leeks, Yellow Rapes, fresh Ragwort roots, confected Sugar, confected Eringo roots, confected Ginger, Costus roots, Sperage, Thistle roots and Radish roots.'[77] While he classed these foods as seed provokers, some were also described elsewhere as full of nourishment, while eryngo, ginger, and others such as radishes were considered to be hot. Others, like stones and 'pissels' were also thought to work through the doctrine of signatures. Aphrodisiacs were thus not consistently separated into different categories by property but might be thought to have multiple properties: they could provoke seed through their heating virtues which also nourished the blood from which seed was produced, or they could also work through the doctrine of signatures, through their resemblance to the organs of generation.

Seed provokers and nourishing foods, like heating foods, continued to be understood as aphrodisiacs throughout the period. Eighteenth-century authors provided their readers with lists of seed provoking aphrodisiacs that were consistent with those from earlier centuries. A particularly extensive list appeared in *Gonosologium novum* (1709), where John Marten wrote that

---

[73] Ibid.
[74] Alessandro Massaria, *De morbis fœminis; the womans counsellor: or, The feminine physitian*, London 1657, 125–30.
[75] Massaria noted that deficient male seed could be a cause of barrenness. It is therefore likely, given his ambiguous gender division of topics, that he thought these were applicable to the male body as well: ibid. 108–12.
[76] Ibid. 126.
[77] Ibid. Massaria also suggested compound recipes that would increase the production of seed.

some particular Foods breed *seed* in all, and are oftentimes found to some People vastly preferable to any sort of Medicines, such as *yolks of Eggs, the Stones of a Cock, Crabbs, Oisters, Lobsters, Cray-fish, Caviar* [sic]*, Marrow, or Pith of Beef Bones, Artichoaks Satyrion-roots, &c.* and above all your large fat silver Eels and their Broth, which beyond all Food raises Lust.[78]

One reason for this consistency was that authors like Marten drew upon earlier works, including Ambrose Paré's surgical treatise. It is consequently not surprising that Marten connected the production of seed not only with sexual stimulation but also with sexual pleasure. Moreover, he suggested that in cases of barrenness these foods were more appealing to patients than other forms of medicine. As in the sixteenth century, seventeenth- and eighteenth-century herbals continued to describe a range of plants that stimulated seed production.[79] One herbal in particular – William Salmon's *Botanologia* (1710) – even included this taxonomy of aphrodisiacs as a type of plant classification in the introduction. Salmon provided a lengthy description of how these substances were thought to affect the body, mentioning both heat and wind as elements participating in their effects:

> SPERMATOGENETICKS. *These are things generating Sperm or Seed. They are hot, and not very dry, but flatulent and spirituous, and breed of the purest and most spirituous parts of the Blood; and therefore all such things as encrease a strong and good Chylus, and from thence much and good Blood, encrease the quantity of the Seed. It is also stimulated by hot, volatil, thin of substance, penetrating and sharp; and hindred by things cold, insipid, non-nutritive, and discutient.*[80]

As is evident here, medical writers were not always clear about how seed provokers stimulated desire and improved fertility, although it was perhaps not necessary to state that more, and better quality, seed was more likely to result in a conception. Several medical texts stated that as seed passed through the body it titillated the genitalia. This process was not straightforward. Seed not only caused pleasure and lust but was also stirred by it, in a complex cyclical relationship; the increasing heat of desire encouraged the body to produce seed ready for ejaculation. Many writers did not debate the complexities of this relationship. Yet some writers did more than simply state that seed was stimulating. The anonymous author of *The compleat doctoress* (1656) wrote that 'Barren men are commonly beardless, slow in imagination, and dull in practise, because their seed is cold, and contains not any spirit to tickle, and warme their Phantasies.'[81] Here it was the heat and spirits

---

[78] Marten, *Gonosologium novum*, 52.
[79] For example see Parkinson, *Theatrum botanicum*, 254–5, 261, 378, 819, 873, 919, 964, 1058, 1136, 1417, 1538; John Pechey, *The compleat herbal of physical plants*, London 1694, 71, 144, 249, 258; and Salmon, *Botanologia*, 100, 263, 265, 325–8, 716–9, 752, 795, 823.
[80] Salmon, *Botanologia*, p. xiii.
[81] Anon., *The compleat doctoress: or, A choice treatise of all diseases insident to women*, London 1656, 131–2.

contained within the seed that increased sexual desire, again highlighting the important relationship between heat, nourishment and the potency of seed. Despite the sometimes ambiguous explanations provided in these texts, it was ubiquitously understood that a body that was not successfully producing seed would fail to feel the pleasure of venereal delights. As is implied above, many authors advocated these substances because they encouraged the body to produce *more* seed than usual. Helkiah Crooke noted that the membranes of the yard were endowed with 'an exquisite sence [sic] to make it capable of the pleasure which the seed in his passage through stirreth up'.[82] Hence, the more seed that passed through the yard the greater the chance of experiencing pleasure.[83] Authors of erotic literature also attested that an abundance of seed caused pleasure, Nicholas Chorier's *Dialogues of Luisa Sigea* (1660) repeatedly drew this connection. For example, one character, Tullia, stated that 'I felt my self drenched with a heavy shower of seed: beneficent Venus had never before caused so copious a shower to fall into my garden. Even now I die of joy … when I think of that hour.'[84] In this instance the amount of seed caused a lasting pleasure that could be easily recalled from memory. Seed-provoking aphrodisiacs were therefore thought to stimulate sexual desire and increase sexual pleasure, which encouraged the orgasm requisite for conception, and encouraged the body to produce potent seed, through the provision of good nourishment, which improved fertility.

Authors like Isbrand van Diemerbroeck believed that seed contained salty particles as well as heat and spirits, which made it stimulating and fertile.[85] Consequently, many early modern medical texts argued that eating salty foods could improve the seed. However, this was not unanimously accepted, and several authors throughout the period contested both the importance of salt, and the use of salty aphrodisiacs. One advocate of salty stimulants was Jacques Ferrand. His treatise discussed love melancholy in both men and women, but in his section describing salt the focus was, as with van Diemerbroeck, on men. He cautioned his readers that the consumption of salty, aromatic and fried foods could lead to love melancholy. He explained that

> Salt, by reason of its Heat and Acrimony, provokes to Lust those that use to eate it in any great quantity. And for this cause the Ægyptian Priests were wont to abstaine from all manner of Salt meats, having found by experience, that salt things doe cause a kind of Itching or Tickling in those parts that serve for Generation.[86]

---

[82] Cooke, *Mikrokosmographia*, 212.
[83] Culpeper, *Culpeper's directory for midwives* (1676 edn), 131.
[84] Chorier, *Luisa Sigea*, 88.
[85] van Diemerbroeck, *The anatomy of human bodies*, 190–1.
[86] Ferrand, *Erotomania*, 245.

Here again heat, provided by the salty particles in the seed, was considered to be a fundamental part of provoking the body to lust and ensuring that seed was potent. He was also clear, in this section at least, that salt merely encouraged sexual activity rather than manifestly improving the fertility of the reproductive organs. Ferrand further argued that this quality was made evident in the natural world. He explained that fishes were more fruitful because they lived in salt water and that shepherds would give salt to their sheep and goats in order to 'awaken in them their Generative Faculty, when it is in a manner quite dulled and dead in them'.[87] The language that Ferrand used here was ambiguous, and could have referred solely to the stimulation of lust, or perhaps more likely given his focus on fecundity that salt made the reproductive organs and seed more fertile. Although the examples that he provided focused on reproduction in animals, their presence in this text was intended to inform readers about the consequences of salt consumption for the human body. Ferrand was expansive in discussing this topic, suggesting that he felt that this was a particularly dangerous group of foods for those wishing to avoid the pricking sensations of lust.

Other medical authors did however pick up on the theme of the acrimonious, salty and brackish nature of seed and foods that could enhance this. Van Diemerbroeck noted that one way in which the salacity of seed could be proved was 'because the increasing of that in quantity excites an itching Titillation, and provoke[s] to Lasciviousness'.[88] Similarly, in the *Mercurius compitalitius* (1684) Theophile Bonet wrote that '*Saline* and *acrimonius* things' were aphrodisiacs 'for as *Venus* is said to be born of the Salt Sea, so saline things do also notably stimulate'.[89] Within this category he suggested that borax (a form of salt crystal) was of particular merit.[90] Like Ferrand before him, Bonet did not stop at a one-line explanation. He continued: 'Likewise such things as are indued with a very biting Salt, that may be melted into the genital Parts, stimulate strongly.'[91] Bonet also hinted at the effects that these salty foods had on the body and, in doing so, expressed again the notion that strong, plentiful, acrimonious and salty seed titillated the generative organs and caused pleasure during intercourse. He stated that 'by the acrimony of the Medicine the seminal vessels may be easily irritated through their vicinity'.[92] Yet the role of salt in seed was not universally accepted. John Marten wrote that 'Some impute the cause of this Pleasure to the Salt of the *Seed* … but I do not believe the *Seed* is possessed of such a quantity of Salts sufficient to prick the Parts through which it passes, and cause such an

---

[87] Ibid. 246. See also Thomas Lupton, *A thousand notable things*, London 1579, 22.
[88] van Diemerbroeck, *The anatomy of human bodies*, 191.
[89] Bonet, *Mercurius compitalitius*, 694.
[90] Ibid.
[91] Ibid.
[92] Ibid.

agreeable Titillation.'[93] Marten did not directly reject the idea that salt stimulated the body. He merely underlined that seed did not contain sufficient quantities of salt for the effects to be felt. Thus, given the wider context in which brackish foods were considered to be aphrodisiacs, this passage could have been interpreted as a further recommendation: consuming salt-based aphrodisiacs would increase the amount of salt in the seed and so make it a more invigorating substance. None of these descriptions explicitly rejected the potential for female seed to be salty, or to need salt in order to be stimulating. However, the focus of nearly all of these authors was on the male body and its seed.

Despite the interpretive scope of Marten's descriptions, the understanding that salty foods were aphrodisiacs was less prominent in eighteenth-century medical literature, unlike the persistent references to aphrodisiacs that heated the body and provided nutrition. As new theories about the generative organs were developed during this period, aphrodisiacs were reassessed. The understanding of these drugs was not static but continually examined and refined. The dismissal of salty foods was possibly influenced by the discovery, by Antoni Leeuwenhoek (and others), of the animalcules (spermatozoa) in male semen in the 1670s. Many eighteenth-century authors discussed the seed, and its potency, in terms which related to the animated and lively motion of the animalcules.[94] This discovery may have overshadowed other ideas such as the role of salt. However, there was a discernible time lapse between this discovery and its subsequent appearance in printed medical treatises. Moreover, a cohesive and unified theory of the seed and its virtues was never achieved in printed works. Some writers continued to mention the acrimony of salt in the 1730s.[95] Nevertheless, the ability of salty foods to increase the titillating quality of the seed was increasingly dismissed, unlike heating and nutritious foods that continued to be advocated throughout the eighteenth century.

Even though there were several ways in which seed-provoking aphrodisiacs were described, it is evident that those writing about these substances did not only recommend them as infertility treatments because they encouraged people to have sex. Seed was the crucial element in producing a conception and so all of these remedies were almost universally understood to promote fertility and encourage conception. In *Dr Chamberlain's midwifes practice* the author explained in the chapter on barrenness that, if nature was dull, 'Remedies to increase Seed, and further Conception in Women,

---

[93] Marten, *Gonosologium novum*, 57–8.
[94] James Keill, *The anatomy of the humane body abridg'd*, London 1718, 116; John Quincy, *Lexicon physic-medicum, or, A new medicinal dictionary; explaining the difficult terms used in the several branches of the profession*, London 1726, 91–2.
[95] John Radcliffe, *Dr. Radcliffe's practical dispensatory, containing a complete body of prescriptions*, London 1730, 192.

and fruitfulnesse in the Seed of Man' should be used.⁹⁶ Although this statement initially appears to be about making men and women aroused, that the author went on to specifically reference conception and fruitfulness shows that he believed that these remedies would do more to make the body fertile. Popular printed materials also suggested that these aphrodisiacs would increase the chances of conception occurring. *Aristoteles master-piece* (1684) recommended seed provokers as the first type of medicament for those who were barren.⁹⁷ The author stated that it was necessary for conception that there was an appetite and desire for copulation and advised that 'if Nature be infeebled, then are there fit artificial Remedies to restore it; *viz*. such meats as most conduce to the affording such aliment as proves to make Seed abound'.⁹⁸ This was followed a few lines later by the recommendation that 'such as are subject to Barrenness should eat such meat only as tend to render them fruitful; and among such things as are inducing and stirring up thereto, are all meats of good juice, that nourish well'.⁹⁹ This author clearly felt not only that provoking the production of seed would cause arousal but that it would improve fertility by making the resultant sex more pleasurable and fruitful. This widely-read tract was reprinted at least fifty times over the eighteenth century, and implies that it was widely understood that seed-provoking aphrodisiacs were a treatment for male and female infertility.¹⁰⁰ The use of nourishing aphrodisiacs to improve both male and female fertility also appeared in some early modern ballads. *The apple-dumpling eater* (1692) extolled the strengthening, or perhaps nourishing, virtues of dumplings, stating that they allowed a man called Rogers to get 'his Wife with Child of Nine Boys at a time'.¹⁰¹ Having recorded the remarkable efficacy of dumplings for strengthening a man's lust and ability to engage in intercourse, the author of the ballad recommended 'You Women that Pray for a Baby,/ Whose Husbands are Feeble and Old,/ Must Eat as much *Dumpling* as may be.'¹⁰² In order for a conception to occur the reproductive body needed to be strong, well-nourished and producing potent seed. This seed would not only stimulate the body to engage in sexual intercourse but would make the resultant sex more pleasurable; the more and better quality seed that passed through the reproductive organs the more stimulated they would become, and because the seed was potent would mean that the ensuing sex was more likely to result in a conception.

[96] Peter Chamberlen, *Dr Chamberlain's midwifes practice*, London 1665, 256.
[97] Anon., *Aristoteles master-piece* (1684 edn), 11.
[98] Ibid.
[99] Ibid.
[100] The English Short Title Catalogue lists versions of *Aristotle's master-piece* appearing at least fifty times between 1700 and 1799. In addition numerous versions were also printed as *Aristotle's last legacy*.
[101] Anon., *The Norfolk stiff-rump: or, The apple-dumpling eater*, London 1692.
[102] Ibid.

Windy meats and flatulent foods

Another group of foods commonly regarded as aphrodisiacs in the medical literature was windy meats, or flatulent foods. These foods were predominantly discussed in relation to the prowess of the male genitalia; their relationship to the female body was not straightforward. Medical authors explained that an erection was caused by blood, imagination, muscles, pressure, seed and wind inflating the penis.[103] Consequently, it was believed that foods which released wind into the body better enabled men to have an erection. To Alessandro Massaria, for example, the strength and stiffness of a man's erection was particularly important in ensuring successful copulation and conception.[104] In this state a man could cast the seed deep into the womb, while it was still warm and potent, thus ensuring a pleasurable sensation, and enhancing the possibility of conception. Furthermore, it was widely acknowledged that a woman's body required more time to become fully stimulated. Hence, a strong, and more importantly, lasting erection facilitated the invigoration of the female generative system, further heating it through the friction of intercourse, allowing it to reach the point where it released its own seed. This enhanced both the pleasurable experience of intercourse and the chances of conception.

Additionally, potent seed was thought to be filled with spirits and wind. There was a long-standing tradition behind this belief. The eleventh-century treatise of Constantine the African noted that ingredients that contained nourishment and a cause of flatulence reproduced the essence of semen: humour and breath.[105] Culpeper's translation of the *Pharmacopoeia londinensis* stated that wind, like heat and salts, was necessary to make seed potent and titillating thus allowing it to stimulate the male reproductive body: 'this faculty [wind] ought to be in Seed, that being heat with spirits it may cause the Yard to stand'.[106] Lævinus Lemnius also argued that the male organs needed to be filled with a 'force of a flatulent spirit, whereby the seed may be driven forth into the Matrix'.[107] Wind thus facilitated successful ejaculation of warm seed into the womb through maintaining an erection and by creating an explosive force of movement. The prompt movement of seed from the testicles to the womb helped to promote conception as the seed lost none of its potency.

Unlike other categories of aphrodisiacs these were thought to be sex-specific. Their effects on the female body were contested and medical prac-

---

[103] Eccles, *Obstetrics and gynaecology*, 36; Crooke, *Mikrokosmographia*, 212.
[104] Massaria, *De morbis fœminis*, 108.
[105] Danielle Jacquart and Claude Thomasset, *Sexuality and medicine in the Middle Ages*, trans. Matthew Adamson, Cambridge 1988, 119.
[106] Culpeper, *Pharmacopoeia londinensis* (1653 edn), 319.
[107] Lemnius, *The secret miracles of nature*, 26.

titioners and the wider populace were not unified in how they recommended their use. Many authors cautioned severely against the use of these foods in women, arguing that wind inside the womb was a damaging condition that could hinder fertility. In the sixteenth century both Jakob Rueff and Philip Barrough cautioned their readers in this way.[108] Barrough specifically warned women that 'windinesse ingendered in the womb, doth let the fertility of conception, & causeth barennesse'.[109] Similarly, in the late seventeenth century, several authors suggested that wind collecting in the womb damaged the reproductive process. This suggests that medical authors increasingly agreed that flatulence was not an element of female fertility or sexual stimulation. Indeed, many writers, including Jane Sharp (1671), offered remedies for removing wind from the womb, as part of their recommendations for curing barrenness.[110] The uncertainty with which medical writers prescribed windy aphrodisiacs to the two sexes implies that medical writers and practitioners did acknowledge that certain aphrodisiacs had to be adapted to suit the sexed body. As Wendy Churchill has argued, medical practice throughout the early modern period was more complex than the one-sex model would allow for; rather it was flexible and took a holistic approach considering the age and sex of the patient as well as their humoural constitution.[111] In this case the inherent differences between the male and female reproductive bodies were acknowledged, and this encouraged medical writers to recognise stimulants that worked specifically on the male generative body. Nonetheless, it should be remembered that substances that were designed to act upon the male generative organs would subsequently have had an impact upon the woman's sexual experience and her ability to conceive.

This 'flatulent' category included beans and peas, which were known as 'windy meats' and, according to Audrey Eccles, were more commonly given to men with hotter constitutions.[112] This may have been because a body that was too hot consumed and burned away the seed, thus destroying sexual pleasure and the chances of conceiving. Therefore, foods not explicitly connected to raising the heat of desire could be safely employed to enhance performance in men of a hot constitution. Nonetheless, although many writers explained that these foods were specifically intended for male patients, this was not always clear. Philip Barrough argued that when a man cannot fulfil his duties 'windie meates are good for him, as be chiche peason, beanes, scallions, leekes, the roote and windy seede of persneppes, pine nuttus, sweet almonde … and other such like'.[113] Barrough described these

---

[108] Rueff cautioned men and women: *The expert midwife*, 48–9.
[109] Barrough, *The methode of phisicke*, 159.
[110] Sharp, *The midwives book*, 176. See also Lemnius, *The secret miracles of nature*, 27.
[111] Churchill, *Female patients*, 176–7.
[112] Eccles, *Obstetrics and gynaecology*, 36; McLaren, *Reproductive rituals*, 34.
[113] Barrough, *The methode of phisicke*, 142.

foods as more effective for men, although they were listed in his section discussing the '*losse of carnall copulation*' in men and women. This lack of clarity may have resulted in the use of these aphrodisiacs by both sexes indiscriminately. In *Erotomania* (1640) Jacques Ferrand listed the types of food found in this category. Although he was not explicit in explaining how they worked, he did suggest that heat, nutrition, flatulence and melancholy all added to their stimulating nature.[114] Ferrand cautioned his readers that to avoid lust 'He must also take heed that he doe not use to eate often, Pine-nuts, Pistachoes, small nuts, Cives, Artichokes, Coleworts, Rapes, Carrots, Parsnips, green Ginger, Erignoes, Satyrion, Onions, Waternuts, Rocket, &c ... Oysters, also, chestnuts, Ciche pease, ... and all such like meats.'[115] Although, for Ferrand, these foods may have contained any one of the key aphrodisiacal elements, there was an overlap with those foods that appeared in Barrough's list: chickpeas, pine-nuts, parsnips and scallions/onions. In a similar manner to other authors Ferrand addressed this list to men, which may have reflected the author's expectation that his audience would be male, or hinted at their sex-specific efficacy.[116]

Herbals in the sixteenth and seventeenth century were similarly explicit in describing windy foods as aphrodisiacs. As with the other genres of aphrodisiacs included in herbals, these descriptions focused almost solely on the fact that these foods would encourage men and women to have sex.[117] Moreover, in herbals, the gender of the potential patient was rarely explicit. As reference works for those using herbs and plants medicinally, including in a domestic setting, they allowed someone to look up the virtues of a particular plant or search for the plants required to treat a specific disorder. They did not, however, always provide in-depth information or present the types of debate seen in more comprehensive medical texts. Consequently they rarely provided details about who should consume particular botanicals: John Parkinson wrote of madde apples (aubergines) only that 'they breed much windinesse, and thereby peradventure bodily lust'.[118] Similarly, Gerard's *Herball* described how dogs stones (a variety of orchis) were full of 'much superfluous windinesse, and therefore being drunke ... stirreth up fleshly lust'.[119] This description would imply that flatulent foods were not sex

---

[114] Ferrand, *Erotomania*, 247.

[115] Ibid. 247–8.

[116] A late seventeenth-century edition of Culpeper's *Directory for midwives* also suggested that men 'eat windy Meats, especially such as nourish much, as Parsneps, Alexanders, Skirrets, Pine-nuts &c' if they experienced a loss of sexual desire: *A directory for midwives*, London 1693, 69.

[117] Turner, *A new herball*, 163; Parkinson, *Theatrum botanicum*, 354, 442, 873, 903, 944, 946, 1076; Gerard, *The generall historie of plantes*, 207, 1026, 1039; Salmon, *Botanologia*, 30–1.

[118] Parkinson, *Theatrum botanicum*, 354.

[119] Gerard, *The generall historie of plantes*, 207.

specific but caused sexual desire, without danger, in both sexes. Thus some readers of these botanical treatises may have assumed that windy aphrodisiacs were suitable for both the male and the female body. Conversely, the authors of these texts may have expected their readers to understand the inherent danger in giving these substances to women. Nonetheless, the lack of clarity in both medical texts and herbals demonstrates that even when aphrodisiac substances were considered to be sex specific this was not asserted with force. The ambivalence of writers in prescribing these particular aphrodisiacs for the male body was also reflected in how they were used in infertility treatments.

Many remedies for female barrenness and infertility across the period included windy meats without any concern about the potential damaging effects that they might have on the female body. The 1676 edition of Nicholas Culpeper's *Directory for midwives* included numerous recipes for combating barrenness.[120] Several of these remedies favoured flatulent, nut-based aphrodisiacs. Yet it is not apparent in these texts that this was because they caused sexual pleasure. One remedy required the consumer to take '*Sweet Almonds, Pistachaes, Pine-Nuts, Hazel-Nuts, each an ounce; Citron Peels, Ginger, Cloves, Cinnamon, each half a dram; Rocket-seed two drams*' and make them into a confection, taken at bedtime.[121] This recipe was intended to 'amend the distemper of the womb' that resulted in no seed or unfruitful seed being produced.[122] Nuts were also thought to be nourishing, which may have allowed for their use in this instance. However, the lack of concern about the use of these aphrodisiacs suggests that many medical writers, and readers, assumed that sexual stimulants were always a useful substance for increasing desire and improving fertility whatever the sex of the patient. Theophile Bonet, unusually, even went as far as to advocate windy substances specifically for the treatment of female barrenness. He did not suggest that they would stimulate sexual desire, but instead advocated them for women whose organs had been closed up by excessive fat.[123] He explained that

> it must be believed that whatever things do dilate, and any way distend the Womb, and lay the Passages of it more open, which are pressed with Fat and the Cawl, are good Medicines for the Womb: which without doubt I think is done by such things as cause Flatulencies, because they are apt to distend the Part where they are.[124]

However, their use in this context may have also facilitated sexual pleasure and conception by allowing the male seed to touch the internal cavity of the

---

[120] Culpeper, *Culpeper's directory for midwives* (1676 edn), 137.
[121] Ibid.
[122] Ibid.
[123] Bonet, *Mercurius compitalitius*, 569.
[124] Ibid.

reproductive organs. It is clear then that medical treatises formed no clear consensus on the stimulating or fertility-enhancing properties of flatulent foods.

The remedies gathered in the manuscript collections of lay men and women also allude to a lack of concern about using windy substances for the treatment of female barrenness. The recipe book of Elizabeth Jacob recorded that 'for Conception', one should 'seeth the fish called A Trout in goats milke, and give it the party to drink when she goes to bed'.[125] Even though the trout was likely to have been the central element of this recipe, the *Pharmacopoeia londinensis* described milk as extremely windy.[126] Recipes where egg whites and milk were gently heated together were also recorded in recipe books attributed to Johanna Saint John and Anne Brockman.[127] Milk was described as an aphrodisiac by a few medical writers, but normally it was associated with nourishing and seed-provoking qualities: for example Alessandro Massaria's *De morbis fœmineis* listed both eggs and milk in a list of medicines that 'encrease natural seed, and stir up venery'.[128] Jacques Ferrand's *Erotomania* did include eggs in a list of aphrodisiacs that were both hot and flatulent, but this appears to be unusual as, again, eggs were associated with nourishment.[129] The use of these substances may therefore simply reflect that they were not strongly associated with breeding wind in the body. However, if these recipe book collectors were aware of the potential for milk to breed dangerous wind in the female body this evidently did not stop them from recommending this type of remedy. Indeed Johanna Saint John's book asserted that this remedy was known to have worked, causing a woman to conceive twice.[130]

The absence of caution about the use of windy aphrodisiacs may have reflected a lack of interest or belief in their effects amongst the wider populace. Seventeenth-century ballads did not readily include windy aphrodisiacs, although one ballad and one humorous pamphlet did include egg-caudles.[131] More commonly, despite its focus on the treatment of male impotence, popular literature included nourishing and warming foods like caudles and cock-broths.[132] Similarly, those popular and erotic texts from the

---

[125] WL, MS 3009, 128.
[126] Culpeper, *Pharmacopoeia londinensis* (1653 edn), 31.
[127] WL, MS 4338, fo. 213v; BL, MS Add. 45197, 59.
[128] Massaria, *De morbis fœminis*, 126; Platter, *A golden practice of physick*, 170.
[129] Ferrand, *Erotomania*, 247.
[130] WL, MS 4338, fo. 213v.
[131] Anon., *The scolding wives vindication*; Anon., *The womans brawl* (title page and date missing), ed. Roger Thompson, in *Samuel Pepys' penny merriments: being a collection of chapbooks, full histories, jests, magic, amorous tales of courtship, marriage and infidelity, accounts of rogues and fools, together with comments on the times*, London 1976, 284
[132] Anon., *The scolding wives vindication*; Anon., *The London cuckold*; Anon., *The sorrowful bride*; Anon., *Labour in vain: or, The taylor no man*, n.p. 1675–96.

period that included aphrodisiacs and remedies to strengthen men's sexual abilities also tended to describe cock-broths and caudles, rather than windy foods, although the *Ten pleasures of marriage* did include eggs in the foods that it described as recommended for barrenness.[133] The divergent opinions expressed in these different genres of texts do not necessarily indicate a contradiction or distinction between popular and elite medicine in the early modern period.[134] Across all levels of society, those studying and practising medicine could draw upon a variety of different medical traditions: astrological, Galenic, Hippocratic, Aristotelian, folkloric and popular and chemical. A person's medical knowledge was therefore determined by the sources of their information, oral knowledge, experience or a variety of medical texts.

Even though medical writers and others recommended recipes that included windy foods, this category of aphrodisiacs was always contested. From the mid-sixteenth century onwards medical writers discussed and criticised the use and effects of these foods. This criticism increased across the seventeenth century, and by the eighteenth century most medical writers overwhelmingly rejected windy meats as aphrodisiacs. One major concern expressed by medical writers was that the efficacy of these substances did not always live up to expectation and that they created an empty sexual experience. In *The secret miracles of nature*, written originally in the mid-sixteenth century, Lemnius recorded that

> Some of our lascivious women will say, that such men that trouble their wives to no purpose, do thunder, but there follows no rain, they do not water the inward ground of the matrix. They have their veins puffed up with wind, but there wants seed.[135]

Although he accepted that wind facilitated an erection, Lemnius emphasised that this was not enough to rectify male infertility as the man still lacked potent seed. The women thus felt cheated, because without the touch of seed the previous sexual activities were rendered unsatisfactory, both in terms of pleasure and the possibility to conceive. As the period progressed, challenges like this became more common and more sustained. By the late seventeenth century Theophile Bonet dismissed the opinions of other medical writers and confidently stated that windy foods were detrimental to the generative body:

> It is commonly reported of Aphrodisiacks, that *Flatus* or wind is necessary to Venery: but though in Boys erection or distension of the *Penis* may seem from

---

[133] Anon., *The crafty whore: or, The mistery and iniquity of bawdy houses laid open*, London 1658, 56; Marsh, *The ten pleasures of marriage* (1682 edn), 77.

[134] Doreen Evenden Nagy, 'Lay and learned medicine in early modern England', in Peter Elmer and Ole Peter Grell (eds), *Health, disease and society in Europe, 1500–1800: a source book*, Manchester–New York 2004, 38–44 at p. 44.

[135] Lemnius, *The secret miracles of nature*, 27.

Flatus, and these may concur by accident, yet they cannot nor ought not to be reckoned among Aphrodisiacks; those things indeed that excite the Spirits stir up Venery, and so make the Seed turgid, but so do not those things that breed or excite wind.[136]

According to Bonet the turgidity of the seed was the important factor in stimulating both arousal and sexual pleasure, but this was not enhanced by the consumption of flatulent foods. In the same manner as Lemnius, Bonet highlighted that wind may have had an effect on the reproductive organs but it did not create or augment seed, and so could not produce desire, pleasure or conception. Similarly, in the eighteenth century, John Marten voiced concerns about the fact that a flatulent erection could result in the emission of 'no *Seed* at all' or through the straining of the vessels an emission of blood.[137] Marten further reasserted these beliefs when advertising his own '*Grand Aphrodisiack or Generative Drops*'.[138] He claimed that his medicines increased the seed and provoked venery, creating a lasting and substantial erection and titillation rather than 'giving bare stimulation or flatulent Erection and Desire as most Provocatives do'.[139] Marten's wording here implied that his aphrodisiac was a suitable treatment for barrenness because it created lasting sensation and pleasure which would encourage conception. Although he suggested that other remedies still imbued the body with wind, by advertising his own remedies in this way he clearly denigrated the ability of windy meats to excite and invigorate the reproductive organs, and in so doing singled out his own remedies as truly effective.

As has been argued throughout this book, many medical writers read, used and in some cases plagiarised existing medical texts. Consequently it is not surprising to find medical writers, who for example read Lemnius' work, rejecting the idea that wind could stimulate the reproductive body. Broader shifts in medical understanding may also have influenced the increasing dismissal of windy foods. In the late seventeenth century medical treatises began to describe the anatomy and erection of the penis as driven by a series of blood vessels: 'being mostly a contexture of Veins, Arteries and Nervous fibres, woven one with another like a Net; and when the Nerves are filled with Animal spirit, and the Arteries with hot and Spirituous blood, then the *Penis* is distended and becomes erect'.[140] In this new model the penis was not an empty gut to be inflated by wind, but was a complex organ filled with nerves and arteries. The promulgation of this new understanding

---

[136] Bonet, *Mercurius compitalitius*, 694–5.
[137] Marten, *Gonosologium novum*, 39. Marten also argued (p. 29) that windy hernias in the testicles caused pain, hindered intercourse and damaged fertility.
[138] Ibid. 49.
[139] Ibid. 49–50.
[140] Gibson, *The anatomy of humane bodies*, 125; Keill, *The anatomy of the humane body abridg'd* (1718 edn), 99; Arnaud de Ronsil, *Plain and easy instructions*, 29.

of the penis's action probably facilitated the dismissal of the role of wind in causing and maintaining an erection. As with salty foods, this debate and controversy illuminates the ways in which medical authors across the period continually questioned and redefined their understanding of sexual stimulants, both which substances were aphrodisiacs and how they affected the body. In this case flatulent foods were increasingly rejected as a stimulant because they did not improve both sexual desire and fertility. While their ability to inflate the penis allowed for intercourse, it did not improve the emission of seed, as heating and nutritious foods did. Consequently, sex stimulated by the consumption of these foods was unlikely to culminate in conception. This empty coition, without the prospect of progeny, was accordingly criticised as unpleasurable.

Sympathetic stimulation and the doctrine of signatures

The aphrodisiacs discussed so far all worked within the Galenic principle of treating diseases and medical disorders with substances of a contrary quality. Thus those who were infertile because of cold, were given hot spices and meats, while those who could not inflate their penises were given windy meats. However, medical writers at this time could draw upon a range of medical theories and frameworks. Consequently, it was also argued that substances could be aphrodisiacs because of their similarity to and sympathy with the reproductive organs. These stimulants were thought to work through hidden (occult) virtues and were identifiable by the outward appearance of the plants and animals from which they were extracted, sometimes referred to as the doctrine of signatures. As they worked through hidden virtues it is not always apparent whether they were only thought to be suitable for infertility because they encouraged sexual desire. However, their use in remedies explicitly designed to promote fertility implies that, as with other aphrodisiacs, they were thought also to improve sexual pleasure, ability and fertility. Sympathetic treatments spread with the ideas of Paracelsus and remained popular across the seventeenth century.[141] Their popularity, though, was not only limited to Paracelsian practitioners. The idea that the book of nature had been inscribed with signs and signifiers had its own ancient heritage and was a part of the heterogeneous medical knowledge of the early modern era.[142] One seventeenth-century medical author, Richard Bunworth, eloquently explained how this premise operated: 'The good and wise Maker of this Universe, hath Created all things after so glorious and beautiful a manner, and hath given to each Creature such an exact comeli-

---

[141] Lynn Thorndike, *A history of magic and experimental science*, VI: *The sixteenth century*, New York–London 1966, 294.

[142] Paula Findlen, 'Empty signs? Reading the book of nature in Renaissance science', *Studies in the History and Philosophy of Science* xxi/3 (1990), 511–18 at pp. 513–15.

ness after its kinde, that there is not any one thing, in the whole world, whose outward lineaments do not truly and justly characterize unto man its inward endowements.'[143] Aphrodisiacs of this kind reflected the sexual nature of the animal from which they came, or, in the case of plants, were endowed with sexual prowess by their phallic appearance. Throughout the period medical authors discussed a variety of substances that provoked lust by their similitude to the genitalia, seed or the promiscuous, virile nature of the animal from which they were taken.

In the sixteenth century Jakob Rueff made particular use of this category of aphrodisiacs in his compound remedies. Although he did not explicitly outline the effects that these aphrodisiacs would have on the generative system, he did state that they would increase desire and improve fertility. He explained that

> It remaineth also to speak a few words of those things which are to be ministred [sic] inwardly, For because the fruitfulnesse of man and wife may be hindred very much for want of desire to be acquainted with Venus, and by impotency and disability of ingendering and effecting Conception, and also by infirmity of the seeds.[144]

Again, Rueff stated that a lack of sexual desire and the infertility of the reproductive organs went hand in hand. The majority of these recipes contained aphrodisiacs by signature. One recipe advised the patient to 'take the stones of a Foxe, Castoreum, the Matrix of a Hare, dryed, of each two drams'.[145] A similar electuary contained 'the Testicles or stones of a Foxe' combined with 'the Braines of Pigeons, Hens, Cocks, Sparrowes, Drakes, Phesans, Stones of a Bull, of a lecherous Goat, of Bore stones ... [and the] dry Pissle of a Bull'.[146] Two distinct characteristics can be identified in the ingredients in these lists: firstly, animal genitalia and, secondly, the brains, although the flesh and genitalia were also consumed, of animals thought to be particularly lascivious.

Male animal genitalia were commonly recommended as aphrodisiacs in a variety of texts. It might be expected that, as they were taken from male animals and reflected the shape and form of human male genitalia, they were only believed to be effective for the male body. As Oswald Croll noted in the introduction to his 1669 treatise 'of Signatures', 'for as the Man and Woman in Nature are distinct, so also should their Remedies be'.[147] However, the genitalia

---

[143] Richard Bunworth, *Homotropia naturae: a physical discourse, exhibiting the cure of diseases by signature*, London 1656, 1–2.
[144] Rueff, *The expert midwife*, 55–6 (irregular pagination).
[145] Ibid. 56. Castoreum is the oily excretion from the testicles of a beaver.
[146] Ibid. 56–7; Conversely Thomas Lupton suggested that a bull's penis would stimulate men but cause a hatred of intercourse in women: *A thousand notable things*, 18–19.
[147] Oswald Croll, *A treatise of Oswaldus Crollius of signatures*, London 1669, sig. A4r (italics original).

of male animals appeared in numerous infertility treatments for both men and women. In the *De morbis foemineis* (1657), a book which focused on treating women, the author included a 'Confection to further fruitfulness in men, and Conception in women' which contained 'bores stones, Stags Pissel, shaven small … (Bulls Pissel if you cannot get the other, will do as well) Sparrows Brains' and numerous other aphrodisiac substances.[148] John Pechey similarly offered a remedy 'to increase Lust, and to help Conception' that included the 'pizzle of a Bull, of the stones of a Hare, or Boar' along with other aphrodisiacs such as eryngo and satyrion.[149] These recipes were primarily designed to encourage fertility but also functioned by bestowing their sexual capabilities upon the genitalia of the consumer to increase sexual pleasure. By enhancing and potentially extending the sexual acts these stimulants allowed the body to increase its natural heat, elaborate and move the seed around the body, and provided time for the woman to become fully aroused and reach orgasm. Furthermore, the fact that animal genitalia were unlikely to have formed a consistent part of the everyday diet suggests that it is the value of their signature that was prized as a treatment for poor sexual function.[150]

The virtues of animal genitalia and lascivious animals were well known amongst the wider populace. Several infertility remedies were recorded in seventeenth-century domestic recipes books that included these aphrodisiacs. Several relatively simple remedies were recorded across two consecutive pages of the book attributed to Jane Jackson.[151] One required the 'braine of a crane' mixed with ganders grease and fox grease,[152] while the other required a 'Harts Codds' and the 'gall of a goate' taken in wine.[153] Each of these ingredients was associated with particularly lecherous creatures, goats and birds, or a particularly potent one, the hart. Again it is evident that the genitals of a male animal were thought to be applicable to the female body. Unlike many other domestic recipe writers Jane Jackson also considered medications applicable to the male body. She recorded two ointments for external application that were designed to aid women's conception by affecting the male organs. The first required the patient to 'take the braine of a crane and medle it with ganders grease and fox grease and keepe it in a vessel of silver or of gould and at what time thou wold have knowledge annoynt therewith they

---

[148] Massaria, *De morbis fœmineis*, 98.

[149] Pechey, *The compleat midwife's practice enlarged*, 320. See also Culpeper, *Culpeper's directory for midwives* (1662 edn), 137.

[150] Alison Sim, *Food and feast in Tudor England*, Stroud 2005, 72–4, 91. Although not applicable to the entire period, Sim suggested that the lower classes ate pottage, bread and home grown fruit and vegetables, while the middling sort also consumed dairy products.

[151] WL, MS 373, fos 73v–74r

[152] Ibid.

[153] Ibid. fo. 74r

yard and shee shall conceave'.[154] The second recipe instructed: 'take juice of satrion that is Cocks pintle and annoynt thy yard and the womans privitie alsoe and strain above powder made of the matrix of a hare and then deale with her, and shee shall conceive'.[155] Both of these recipes contained aphrodisiacs by signature which were expected to increase a man's sexual potency and prowess. It is thus likely that they were being recommended because they enhanced the pleasure and fertility of the encounter, not because they prompted the men and women to it; enhancing the man's sexual abilities would have encouraged lasting intercourse, allowing a woman the time needed to become stimulated enough to release her seed. The second remedy would also have been designed directly to stimulate the female genitalia, thus increasing the chances of both seeds being emitted and mingling to form a foetus. The continued presence of women in these recipes, the fact that the remedies are to be given to both partners and that they are to make the woman conceive, suggests that many medical practitioners still accepted that infertility was a predominantly female disorder, particularly where the man was able to achieve an erection and ejaculation. However, referring to the woman's body and fertility in these recipes could also have served to conceal a deficiency on the man's part; he could participate in a treatment for his wife without having to acknowledge the remedy's effects upon his own body. That the same recipe was thought to affect both partners simultaneously also suggests a continued acceptance of the similarities between men's and women's bodies into the mid-seventeenth century.

Aphrodisiacs by signature also appeared relatively frequently in ballads, pornographic literature and jests. In *The womans brawl* the protagonist Doll complained:

> Thou unnatural clown thou, feeble Dick thou: As I am Honest Woman Neighbour (I went like a fool) and made him a Caudle with Turkey-eggs, and afterwards a Tanzey with new-laid eggs, from a Hen trod by a Game Cock, put in comfrey and Clary, and fed him Lamb-stones, cavior, and potatoe-pies: yet he could do no more good to a woman then a Boy of a year old.[156]

As in this story, lamb-stones also appeared in *The sorrowful bride* and the *Scolding wives vindication*.[157] Although lamb-stones were widely believed to improve a man's potency and increase a woman's chances of conceiving, medical writers did not describe them as an aphrodisiac, probably because they came from a pre-pubescent animal that would not be renowned for its

---

[154] Ibid. fos 73v, 74r
[155] Ibid. fo. 74r. See also BL, MS Sloane 2485, fo. 48r.
[156] Anon., *The womans brawl*, 284.
[157] Anon., *The sorrowful bride*; Anon., *The scolding wives vindication*.

sexual potency.¹⁵⁸ This divergence of opinion implies not that early modern men and women misunderstood medical theory, but that ideas were adapted to fit with common circumstances: the understanding of animal genitalia as stimulating was applied to a foodstuff – lamb – that, following the Enclosure Acts, was increasingly eaten by families.¹⁵⁹ Similar sentiments appeared in the seventeenth-century pornographic work *The crafty whore*. In this publication a notorious, manipulative prostitute attempted to be faithful to one husband.¹⁶⁰ To try to make her husband more sexually aroused and to improve the pleasure of their encounters, making him a match for her own insatiable lusts, she 'very often gave him caudles, cock-broth, Lamb-stones, &c'.¹⁶¹ In both of these stories the use of these aphrodisiacs failed. This failure played upon early modern ideas about the voracious sexual appetites of women who could be consumed with lasciviousness, in particular the prostitute in *The crafty whore* who, used to copulation with many men while plying her trade, could not be satisfied by her husband alone. Against such appetites, these stories suggested, aphrodisiacs were simply not strong enough to render a husband capable of satisfying his wife. The use of this narrative trope in both of these genres may imply that the populace of early modern England were actually ambivalent about aphrodisiacs, believing that they could be efficacious and suitable to treat infertility, but also easily dismissed as ineffective and unable to strengthen the sexual and reproductive capabilities of impotent men.

It was not only animal genitalia that were considered to be aphrodisiacs; many game birds were also thought to be stimulating. The meat of these birds was hot and nourishing. To restore sexual desire Philip Barrough advocated 'the flesh of hennes, capons, patrich, feasantes, yong doves, birdes of mountains, and specially sparrowes' for their heating and nutritive value.¹⁶² However, these birds were also considered to be prone to lasciviousness: in the 1651 edition of the *Directory for midwives* Nicholas Culpeper stated that '*whatsoever any Creature is addicted extreamly to, they move the man that eats them, to the like* ... therefore Partridges, Quails, Sparrows, &c. being exceeding addicted to Venery, they work the same in those men and women that eat them'.¹⁶³ The belief that sparrows in particular were lecherous had a long pedigree: in Latin 'sparrow' was a synonym for penis.¹⁶⁴ Again, this emphasises that aphrodisiacs were often understood to promote sexual desire

---

¹⁵⁸ Ram's stones were mentioned occasionally. *Aristotle's manual of choice secrets* did include lamb-stones as remedy for barrenness: Anon., *Aristotle's manual of choice secrets, shewing the whole mystery of generation*, London 1699, 132.
¹⁵⁹ Joan Thirsk, *Food in early modern England*, London 2007, 237.
¹⁶⁰ Anon., *The crafty whore*, 56.
¹⁶¹ Ibid.
¹⁶² Barrough, *The methode of phisicke*, 142. See also Platter, *A golden practice of physick*, 170.
¹⁶³ Culpeper, *A directory for midwives* (1651 edn), 88.
¹⁶⁴ McLaren, *Impotence*, 4.

and fertility in several ways. It was not necessarily important for their exact effects to be explained. In the medical literature from across the period there was a common understanding about which animals were considered to be particularly libidinous, and thus could be consumed as aphrodisiacs. In addition to small birds and game, stags, bulls, boars and goats were also considered in this way. Indeed, 'goat' was used in the seventeenth century, as it is today, to describe lecherous and lascivious men.[165] Thus, Jakob Rueff advised that the brains of 'a lecherous Goat' be included in an electuary for improving sexual drive and ability.[166] The sexual prowess of the stag made its horns, also phallic in shape, and its genitalia particularly potent.[167] The epitome of this understanding was the belief that substances taken from these animals while they were engaged in sexual activity were the most potent: the general medical treatise of John Pechey explained that 'the Horns of a Bull rasped is reckoned good for Impotents, especially if it be rasped off in the Time of Coition; so is also the Brain of a Sparrow killed in Coition'.[168] Likewise Theophile Bonet explained that 'the sperm of a Stag killed in *Coition* is a great *arcanum* to provoke *Venus*'.[169] This was likely because at this point the seed had been elaborated to its most refined and pleasurable state and so would incite the greatest amount of sexual pleasure in the consumer.

Philippa Pullar has suggested that several plants were also considered to be stimulating because of their phallic shape, including carrots and parsnips.[170] Although there is little evidence in the medical and herbal literature of this association, carrots and parsnips were frequently described as aphrodisiacs because they were both nutritious and windy. Yet the long-standing history of the doctrine of signatures may have made these discussions superfluous. Laurence Totelin has drawn attention to the presence of numerous phallic vegetables in the original Hippocratic corpus of gynaecological recipes.[171] Thus it could be that for medical writers and practitioners well versed in the knowledge of the ancient medical authorities, the nature and virtue of many phallic plants did not require any explanation. An eighteenth-century erotic text also hinted that carrots and parsnips were stimulating because of

---

[165] *OED*, *s.v.* 'goat', accessed 10 July 2013. The sources do not specify that the goats being discussed are male, but this can be inferred as the others are all the male versions of the animal.

[166] Rueff, *The expert midwife*, 56–7; Croll stated that the yards of bulls and harts excited the venereal faculty because the animals were lascivious: *A treatise of signatures*, 19.

[167] The sexual nature of deer was described by Aristotle: Laurence Totelin, 'Sex and vegetables in the Hippocratic gynaecological treatises', *Studies in History and Philosophy of Science, part C: Studies in History and Philosophy of Biological and Biomedical Sciences* xxxviii/3 (2007), 531–40.

[168] John Pechey, *A plain introduction to the art of physic*, London 1697, 200.

[169] Bonet, *Mercurius compitalitius*, 546.

[170] Pullar, *Consuming passions*, 237.

[171] Totelin, 'Sex and vegetables'.

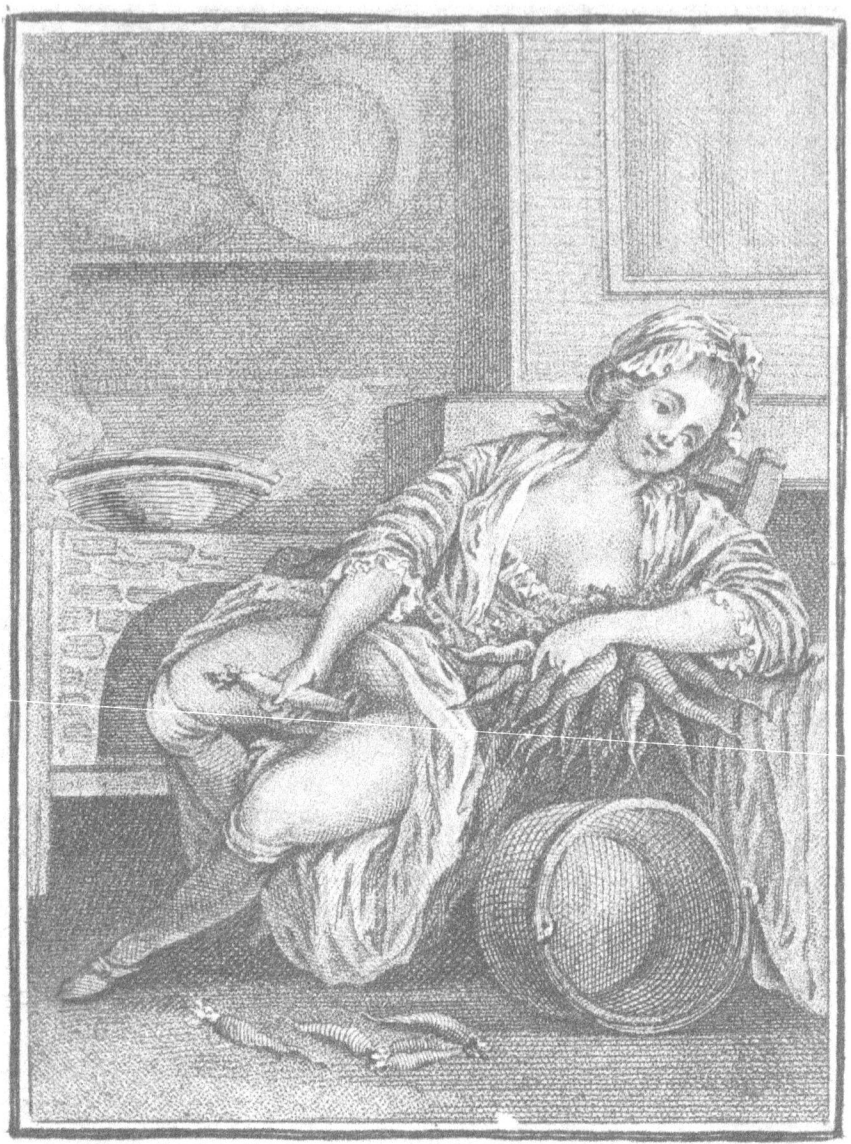

Figure 2. Illustration of a woman masturbating in a kitchen from Samuel Cock, *A voyage to Lethe*, London 1741, unpaginated (©The British Library, London, Cup.1001.c.4)

their shape: an engraving inserted into *A voyage to Lethe* portrayed a woman in a kitchen masturbating with either a carrot or a parsnip (*see* Figure 2).[172] Not only did this highlight the phallic nature of the plant but may also have suggested to readers that aphrodisiac vegetables such as these made particularly good dildos because they were inherently stimulating. Oswald Croll's treatise on the doctrine of signatures argued that, in addition to resembling the entire penis, some plants, notably beans and acorns, also resembled the glans of the penis.[173] Croll did not suggest that this made beans an aphrodisiac, but readers of William Salmon's *Botanologia* (1710) were informed that a strong broth of beans stirred up lust and was good for 'Impotency in the Male Kind, who have not the power to use the Act of Generation' both because it was nutritious and 'by reason the *Bean*, (especially the Field Kind) has the Signature of the *Glans* of the *Penis*, *Pythagoras* and his Followers judged then [sic] to provoke Lust'.[174]

The signature that was most often described by medical and herbal writers was resemblance to the testicles. In the seventeenth century the *Golden practice of physick* informed readers that some stimulants worked through 'their secret hidden quality which was observed by the first teachers of such things, from the whiteness of the flesh, fruits and roots, resembling seed: Or, because taken from Lecherous Creatures; Or from their shape resembling Stones'.[175] Although the authors of a *Golden practice of physick* did not provide any specific examples of foods that resembled seed, they did state that mushrooms and toad-stools were aphrodisiacs because they looked 'like a rough wrinkled Cod'.[176] Oswald Croll included a chapter on the plants that resembled the stones or genitalia, separately from a chapter on those things that resembled the penis, in his book on the doctrine of signatures, most of which he described as 'exciters of the Venerial Faculty'.[177] The focus on plants with the appearance of testicles, which produced seed, and to a lesser extent seed itself, reinforces the central role of seed to both the processes of sexual pleasure and conception.

The first plant type that Croll discussed in this chapter was orchis.[178] These plants were widely discussed in medical and herbal literature as particularly potent aphrodisiacs. Many of the varieties were named, in both Latin and English, after their resemblance to the male genitalia: dogs stones

---

[172] Samuel Cock, *A voyage to Lethe*, London 1741.
[173] Croll, *A treatise of signatures*, 5.
[174] Salmon, *Botanologia*, 79.
[175] Platter, *A golden practice of physick*, 170.
[176] Ibid. Francis Bacon also described mushrooms as aphrodisiacs but for their windiness: *Sylva sylvarum: or, A naturall history in ten centuries written by the right honorable Francis Lo. Veralum Viscount St. Alban: published after the authors death, by William Rawley doctor of divinitie, late his lordships chaplain*, London 1627, 140.
[177] Croll, *A treatise of signatures*, 5–6.
[178] Ibid. 5.

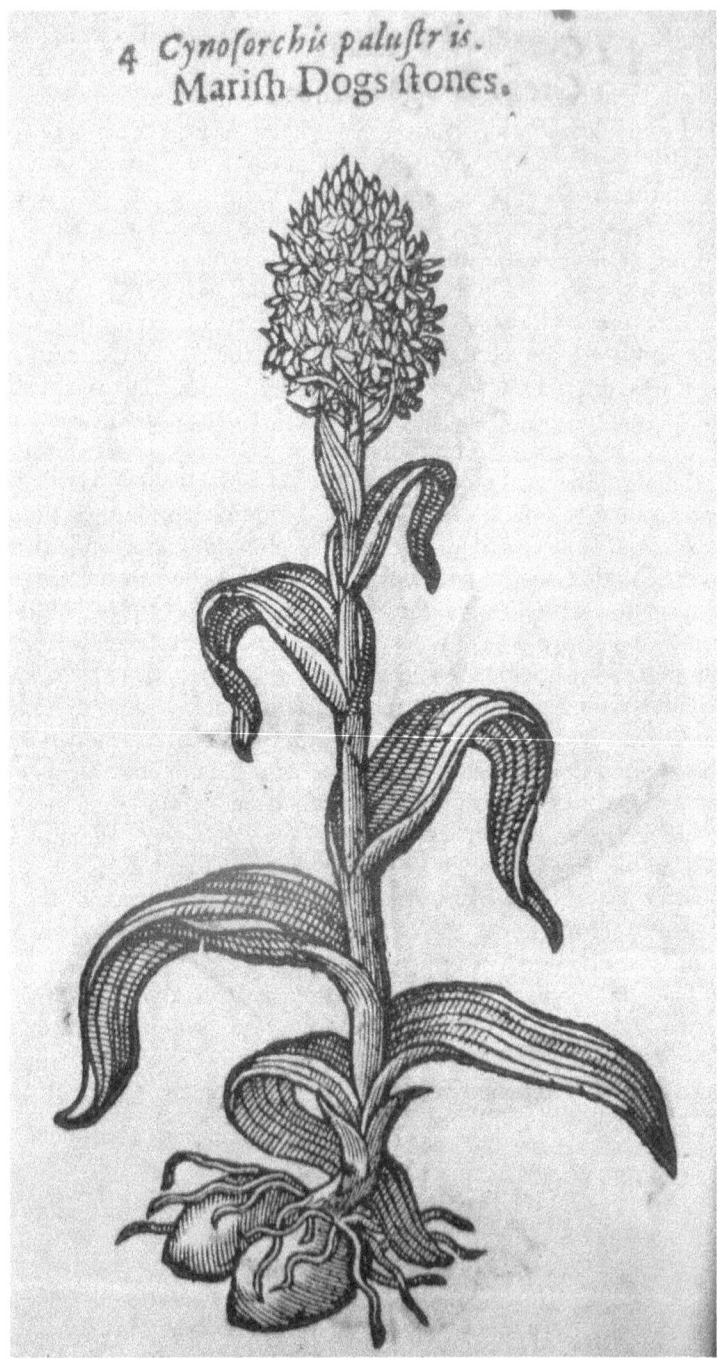

Figure 3. Illustration of Marish dog stones from John Gerard, *The herball or generall historie of plantes*, London 1633 (Archbishop Marsh's Library, Dublin)

(testiculos caninos), fools stones (testiculos morionis), fox stones (testiculos vulpinos).[179] The most frequently mentioned of these was satyrion, sometimes also called dog-stones, which attained a particular renown as an aphrodisiac in the early modern period.[180] Indeed Croll thought that this was so potent that it provoked lust 'being only held in the Hand'.[181] In his work on curing illness through the doctrine of signatures Richard Bunworth only mentioned one aphrodisiac: 'The Roots of *Satyrion*, or Doggs-stones, represent the Testicles in figure, and are famous for their extimulation to venery.'[182] The aphrodisiac qualities of this plant were noted in various genres of text. Numerous herbals described satyrion and other orchis types as aphrodisiacs, although some attributed this not to the erect fleshy stem and accompanying testicular roots of these plants but to their heating and nutritive qualities.[183] Nonetheless, several of these authors noted that the firm roots or full and sappy roots were better for this purpose than those that were loose, soft or spongy. The drawings that accompanied these descriptions also clearly highlighted the perceived similarity to the male genitalia, with an erect stem and bulbous roots covered in tiny hairs (*see* Figure 3). Satyrion also appeared in erotic literature. In *The practical part of love* (1660), a salacious text detailing the extravagant and lascivious life of a prostitute and her daughter, the author suggested that by employing this root a person could reignite an 'almost extinguished and decayed lechery'.[184]

This plant's reputation was also enduring; writers in the late seventeenth and eighteenth centuries continued to describe it as an aphrodisiac. Theophile Bonet suggested that it acted to provoke lust because it was 'slippery and frothy' like the character of seed.[185] This may represent a shift in the way in which this plant was supposed to work, moving from just encouraging sexual activity to making the seed potent, pleasurable and fertile. This again demonstrates the malleability with which definitions and characteristics could be applied to stimulating materials. In this case the satyrion was identified not for its resemblance to the testes but to what they produced. In the eighteenth century John Marten still confidently asserted that the root

---

[179] Parkinson, *Theatrum botanicum*, 1343.

[180] Platter, *A golden practice of physick*, 170.

[181] Croll, *A treatise of signatures*, 6. Pullar commented that the Romans also believed the same: *Consuming passions*, 238.

[182] Bunworth, *Homotropia naturae*, 48.

[183] Rembert Dodoens, *A niewe herbal*, London 1578, 222–5; Newton, *Approoved medicines*, 60; Turner, *A new herbal*, 157; Gerard, *Generall historie of plantes*, 207, 219; Salmon, *Botanologia*, 1010.

[184] Anon., *The practical part of love extracted out of the extravagant and lascivious life of a fair but subtle female*, London 1660, 51. The daughter of the prostitute uses satyrion and eryngo root to renew her failing nature while on a walk through a garden of virtuous plants.

[185] Bonet, *Mercurius compitalitius*, 694.

'given in Wine, does powerfully excite *Venus*' but, unlike previous authors, he did not overtly refer to the doctrine of signatures in his explanation.[186] Instead Marten merely described the importance of the root's colouring: it needed to be red on the outside and white on the inside.[187] Even though this particular description made no allusion to the shape of the plant or its frothy nature, the imagery used by Marten could still be interpreted as an implicit reflection, or retention, of the doctrine of signatures. Readers may have related the red and the white colouring to the flesh colour of the testicles and the white seed that they would have expected to find within. Moreover, this description closely resembled that provided in 1669 by Oswald Croll: '*Satyrion Erythronium*, that is, red *Satyrion*, the exteriour Rinde of the Root is pleasingly red, but within it is white: it as powerfully excites Lust.'[188] Despite the small degrees of difference with which satyrion root was described, it was recognised as one of the foremost aphrodisiacs available in early modern England.

As with the other aphrodisiacs discussed in this chapter, satyrion appeared in medical texts as an ingredient in fertility remedies, or simply recommended by itself. It was, for example, an ingredient in Alessandro Massaria's 'Confection to further fruitfulness in Men, and Conception in Women' as well as in a confection to increase seed and cure barrenness.[189] Similarly, candied satyrion appeared in Lazarus Riverius' first remedy designed to help conception and 'procure desire of fleshly Imbracements'.[190] In this context its reputation was similarly enduring: Robert Johnson's *Praxis medicinae reformata* (1700) informed its readers that infertile men and women should 'make use of those things which have a peculiar virtue to help or cause Conception, and remove Barrenness' including the roots of satyrion.[191] Satyrion thus achieved a notoriety that related to its dual ability to excite sexual stimulation and to improve fertility by improving the pleasurable nature of seed.

This notoriety, however, was not always explicitly tied to the doctrine of signatures. By the seventeenth century this poetic and philosophical approach to understanding nature was under attack from those who claimed that it was a fantasy of idle minds.[192] It was suggested that the sheer number of signs reproduced in the natural world meant that they were inherently unstable

---

[186] Marten, *Gonosologium novum*, 46.
[187] Ibid.
[188] Croll, *A treatise of signatures*, 6.
[189] Massaria, *De morbis foeminis*, 98, 127 (irregular pagination). For other examples see George Hartman, *The true preserver and restorer of health*, London 1682, 292; Pechey, *The compleat midwife's practice*, 317, 320; Wirtzung, *The general practice of physicke*, 300; and Hannah Woolley, *The accomplish'd lady's delight in preserving, physick, beautifying and cookery*, London 1675, 143.
[190] Riverius, *The practice of physick*, 507.
[191] Johnson, *Praxis medicinae reformata*, 247.
[192] Findlen, 'Empty signs?', 517.

and not useful.[193] Medical writers continued to discuss sympathetic remedies for infertility. However, the minor changes in the descriptions provided of satyrion across the early modern period shows how this understanding of medicines was beginning to fade from mainstream thought, leaving a selection of renowned aphrodisiacs to be listed by name alone. These may have persisted because of the commendations of previous authors and as a result of experience. By the late eighteenth century William Smith was writing of the difficulties associated with identifying the actions of certain medications.[194] Those aphrodisiacs that functioned by the doctrine of signatures, without necessarily inducing recognisable results such as seed stimulation, may have been subject to this kind of scrutiny. The decreasing discussion of their attributes means that in later texts it is difficult to assess the degree to which the doctrine of signatures was sustained. Nonetheless, it is clear that medical authors continued to recommend the use of satyrion and aphrodisiacs based upon animal genitalia into the eighteenth century.

Throughout this chapter, it has been observed that a large number of aphrodisiacs and infertility remedies that contained aphrodisiacs were not prescribed for the treatment of a particular sex. Moreover, even when certain remedies were recommended specifically for male or female infertility, they could still contain aphrodisiac ingredients that were considered to be useful to the reproductive body regardless of sex. Nonetheless, this unsexed approach to aphrodisiacs and the treatment of barrenness and impotence should not be overstated. Many midwifery manuals, due to their subject matter, focused on the female body. Similarly some medical writers did include sex-specific remedies for men: Theophile Bonet outlined several aphrodisiacs designed to stimulate the male body in his chapter on '*Leachery and Impotency*', including his claim that 'if the right great Toe be anointed with Oyl in which *Cantharides* have been dissolved it will cause an admirable erection'.[195] *Aristotle's master-piece* also included male-specific aphrodisiacs that contained 'a power to accumulate or heap up Seed, as also to augment it; and other things of force to cause Erection'.[196] However, this may be because, attributed as it was to Aristotle, this work subscribed to the Aristotelian one-seed model of generation in which only men contributed seed to conception. Its remedies to provoke the seed were therefore clearly aimed at men. By contrast, in other works that subscribed to the Galenic-Hippocratic two-seed model, seed-provokers were treatments equally relevant for both men and women. It is evident therefore that medical writers were able to focus on male and female bodies separately if required, while drawing upon

---

[193] Ibid. 518.
[194] William Smith, *Nature studied with a view to preserve and restore health: containing an explanation of the animal oeconomy*, London 1774, 85.
[195] Bonet, *Mercurius compitalitius*, 545–6.
[196] Anon., *Aristotle's master-piece* (1694), 7.

a medical framework and understanding of aphrodisiacs that was applicable to both sexes.

Overall the broadly consistent unsexed nature of these medicaments consequently suggests that even though medical theory and bodily anatomy during the early modern period favoured a two-sex model of the reproductive body this was not necessarily reflected in medical treatments. Medical writers were after all attempting to promote their own services and remedies; they were therefore likely to draw upon a range of ideas, both new and old, in order to appeal to a broad customer base. The way in which infertility was discussed and treated leads us to a more nuanced understanding of early modern medical theory than is offered by arguing for the dominance of either the 'one-sex' or 'two-sex' model. It is evident that medical writers could discuss aphrodisiacs that were sexed and specific only to the male body. However, it is equally evident that for the most part aphrodisiacs were universal; they were believed to be effective in both the male and female bodies without distinction. This supports Churchill's belief that remedies and medicines could be un-sexed but that medical practice was more complex, and could involve sexed treatment plans when and where necessary.[197] However, it does not support the idea that early modern medical practice was fundamentally sexed in its treatment of all diseases. The use of aphrodisiacs was predominantly un-sexed and they were almost universally considered to be suitable treatments for both male and female infertility. It is consequently important to reconsider the drive towards histories of infertility, and other women's health topics, as solely about women's bodies and women's agency. Female infertility cannot be separated from male impotence or infertility, and women's experiences of these issues were intimately connected to male experiences and involved male actors. Fundamentally, the treatment of the infertile and reproductively dysfunctional body was not defined by sex, but by the convictions that the sexually driven and pleasurable body was a procreative body, and that procreative sex was inherently more pleasurable.

The consistent connection between sexual pleasure and conception in discussions of aphrodisiacs in medical texts between 1550 and 1780 also complicates the argument that erotic sexuality was gradually disassociated from reproduction during the eighteenth century: what has been described as the first sexual revolution. Thomas Laqueur, for example, argued that 'sexual pleasure and the whole gigantic apparatus of desires, institutions, and restraints that had for so long been linked almost entirely to reproduction began to become unmoored'.[198] Similarly Faramerz Dabhoiwala has shown

---

[197] Churchill, *Female patients*, 177.
[198] Thomas Laqueur, 'The rise of sex in the eighteenth century: historical context and historiographical implications', *Signs* xxxvii/4 (2012), 802–12 at p. 810.

that the regulation of sexuality in the seventeenth century was rooted in the teachings that '[l]ust was a dangerous and shameful passion, that fornication was evil' and that adultery was criminal.[199] From this basis the social, political and religious changes of the late seventeenth and eighteenth centuries paved the way for more liberated attitudes to sexuality. From a religious and legal perspective on the regulatory attitude of the seventeenth century this was certainly true, but if we incorporate medical understandings of licit sexual activity into this narrative we gain a much more nuanced picture. Medical texts offered a discourse on the legitimate role of sexual desire and pleasure by demonstrating its God-given role in generation. They demonstrate that for early modern men and women sex was 'sexy' because it was reproductive; sexual pleasure and procreation were inextricably linked in the medical doctrines prevalent in society from the sixteenth through to the later eighteenth centuries. Aphrodisiacs continued to link sexual pleasure and reproduction throughout the era. Thus attitudes towards sexuality were likely to have been more complex than simply viewing illicit sexual behaviours as more pleasurable and freer from the constraints of generation. Desire and pleasure could be experienced in a range of settings and contexts including legitimate, marital, generative sexual encounters.

Finally, although much of what has been described here could be regarded as theoretical discussion, it is worth remembering that the loss of sexual desire, the inability to reproduce and the consequent use of aphrodisiacs were very real and very distressing issues for some early modern men and women. Isbrand van Diemerbroeck recorded in his observations of medical practice that this was a problem for which people sought and received medical help. In response to such a request van Diemerbroeck emphasised that medical practitioners, and perhaps others, turned to a combination of aphrodisiac substances and virtues in order to strengthen both potency and fertility. He described how having treated a man for a festered splinter in his thigh,

> The Country-man complained to me of another Malady no less ungrateful to his Wife, that his Inclinations to conjugal performance were utterly extinguish'd, and his Venereal Ability quite lost, which Malady he said had befallen him but since the Cure of his Thigh. Presently I suspected that this Languidness proceeded from the use of the Camphire, which I had mixed with the Balsam and other Plaisters; so that I forbore the farther use of it, and gave the Country-man Electuary of Dyasatyrion to take, and prescrib'd him a Nourishing Dyet of Hot Meats, with Spices, Leeks and Onions, which restored him to that Degree that he followed his Wives *Agriculture* as he was wont to do.[200]

---

[199] Dabhoiwala, *The origins of sex*, 24.
[200] van Diemerbroeck, *The anatomy of human bodies*, 79 (irregular pagination).

It was through the use of aphrodisiacs that this man recovered his desire for intercourse and his ability to satisfy his wife. In using the common agricultural metaphor van Diemerbroeck also informed the readers of this text that aphrodisiacs had restored the potential for this couple to conceive children.

4

Enchanted Privities and Provokers of Lust

Readers of the English edition of Mattheus Gottfried Purmann's surgical treatise (1706) were regaled with the story of a twenty-eight old year clothier, whose penis had swelled with water, making it difficult for him to urinate and to engage in sexual activity with his new wife.[1] Purmann wrote of this unfortunate man that 'the Patient would not be perswaded but his Wife had *Bewitch'd* him'.[2] He described how the patient received treatment that released the water from his swollen genitalia and returned everything to its natural proportion:

> Thus he continued three Weeks together, and as it may be guessed made use of his Young Wife as formerly; whereupon the swelling returned as before, and to add to his Affliction, he was again tormented with the apprehension that his Wife had bewitched him, and would not be perswaded to the contrary, by all the Arguments we could use against so Foolish an Opinion.[3]

The clothier died after receiving further treatment.[4] Although this observation was ostensibly about a watery swelling, it is clear that this patient turned to witchcraft to explain his inability to engage in sexual intercourse – his resumption of these activities following his first treatment suggests that he had been unable to do this prior to seeing the surgeon. What is also evident from this case is that the medical practitioners from whom he sought help did not acknowledge bewitchment as a reason for his ailments. Moreover, they were frustrated by the clothier's reluctance to accept the natural nature of his problems.

This clothier was not alone; many in early modern Europe believed that witchcraft posed a threat to their bodies and physical well-being. The Bible provided substantial evidence that witchcraft and demonic interference in the world were real. It was widely acknowledged in medical writings and other texts that God gave the devil the ability to cause reproductive failure. Cases of impotence magic were rare in England. Only two cases were published: the case of Frances Howard and Robert Devereux, third

---

[1] Mattheus Gothofredus Purmannus, *Chirurgia curiosa: or, The newest and most curious observations and operations in the whole art of chirurgery*, London 1706, 144. The story is dated 1694.
[2] Ibid.
[3] Ibid.
[4] Ibid.

earl of Essex, and the bewitching of the earl of Rutland and his wife by the Flowers family. However, it is apparent that on a theoretical level there was concern about this kind of *maleficium*. Moreover it is evident that when medical writers, such as Purmann, were confronted with readers and patients who believed that witchcraft and diabolical intervention were the cause of their reproductive and sexual disorders, they encouraged the idea that the proper response to these ailments, alongside prayer, was to employ a natural remedy. In particular, medical writers emphasised the efficacy of aphrodisiacs in curing sterility of this nature.

Many historians have investigated the relationship between religion, magic and healing. Keith Thomas and Alan Macfarlane both suggested that there were large numbers of cunning folk in this period and that employing their services for cures was common in cases of bewitchment resulting in illness.[5] Thomas's suggestions were subsequently critiqued as scholars explored differing aspects of magical healing.[6] The popularity and origins of cunning folk, and the relationship between popular ideas of magic and the Church, have also been explored by social and cultural historians.[7] Scholars have also investigated the views of medical practitioners on illness caused by witchcraft and recourse to popular magic for its treatment. Yvonne Petry has highlighted that the involvement of medical writers in discussing magically-induced illness meant that they were a part of the great intellectual endeavour of the early modern period – to clarify the boundaries between the natural and the supernatural.[8]

The conclusions that medical writers came to about natural and supernatural illness were varied. Charles Webster has shown that the Protestant-influenced views of Paracelsus claimed that any healing which appeared magical was in fact enacted through natural means.[9] Alternatively David Gentilcore has demonstrated that in Counter-Reformation Italy ideas about bewitchment were complex, with some physicians admitting the powerlessness of natural remedies while others promoted the efficacy of natural remedies in these situations.[10] Petry has noted that medical writers and practitioners tended to seek a natural explanation if one were available, but

---

[5] Keith Thomas, *Religion and the decline of magic*, London 1991, 209–23; Alan Macfarlane, *Witchcraft in Tudor and Stuart England: a regional and comparative study*, London 1999, 115–21.

[6] Ronald Sawyer, '"Strangely handled in all her lyms": witchcraft and healing in Jacobean England', JSH xxii/3 (1989), 461–85 at p. 462.

[7] Owen Davies, *Cunning-folk: popular magic in English history*, London 2003; Euan Cameron, *Enchanted Europe: superstition, reason, and religion, 1250–1750*, Oxford 2010.

[8] Yvonne Petry, 'Many things surpass our knowledge: an early modern surgeon on magic, witchcraft and demonic possession', SHM xxv/1 (2012), 47–64 at p. 47.

[9] Charles Webster, 'Paracelsus confronts the saints: miracles, healing and the secularization of magic', SHM viii/3 (1995), 403–21 at p. 412.

[10] David Gentilcore, *Healers and healing in early modern Europe*, Manchester 1998, 22–5.

that they acknowledged the ability of the devil to interfere with health.[11] Moreover, she has argued that physicians, in a bid to discredit irregular practitioners, affirmed the existence of demonic magic; they then upheld their own knowledge and learning as the only means of discerning a natural from a preternatural illness.[12] This chapter contributes to this complex picture by discussing medical responses to infertility magic. Angus McLaren has argued that sympathetic and ritualistic cures were commonly used in cases of impotence magic in England and France throughout the seventeenth century.[13] Similarly, Edward Muir noted in *Ritual in early modern Europe* that impotence magic was initially combated with ritualistic responses, such as making urine through the wedding ring or through the door of the church in which the man was married.[14] Later in the period it became more common to seek the blessing of a priest or minister to remove the spell. Although these methods of removing infertility magic were certainly discussed by English demonologists and writers on witchcraft, investigations into these responses has tended to focus on continental Europe. This chapter will consider how medical texts published and read in England described this problem, its causes and its cures. It will be shown, as Webster, Gentilcore and Petry have implied, that many medical writers believed that illness of this kind could be combated by employing natural cures. They sought to delineate and promote the efficacy of natural remedies in their texts, and this formed a core aspect of the response to infertility enchantments alongside the healing provided by the clergy. The use of aphrodisiacs in the context of preternatural illness and religious beliefs underlines that these substances were crucial to remedying a range of different types of infertility in the early modern period. Moreover, it demonstrates that, in cases of impotence magic, provoking lust in order to make sure that husbands and wives engaged in sexual activity was central to understanding their use and function. Aphrodisiacs re-invigorated the libido to enable it to overcome enchantments and spells that dampened it and strengthened the reproductive organs and seed to increase the chances of a conception occurring, which would prove definitively that magic of this kind had been removed.

Witchcraft, spells and enchantments

Medieval discussions of magic, diabolism and witchcraft were instrumental in shaping the ideas of scholars and the wider populace in the early modern period. Richard Kieckhefer has outlined how the intellectual elites of

---

[11] Petry, 'Many things surpass our knowledge', 48.
[12] Ibid. 50.
[13] McLaren, *Impotence*, 52.
[14] Edward Muir, *Ritual in early modern Europe*, Cambridge 2005, 46–7.

medieval Europe acknowledged two broad strands of magic, natural and demonic.[15] Natural magic dealt with the hidden or occult virtues of natural things, demonic magic involved the perversion of religious rituals to appeal to demonic forces for help in human affairs.[16] Within medieval texts the devil's power to affect the body and specifically the reproductive organs was often debated. Authors questioned the nature of this power and the devil's methods. The *Malleus maleficarum [The hammer of the witches]*, written by Heinrich Kramer and James Sprenger and dated to 1487, declared that even though the devil did not damage the reproductive organs, he could render them useless and remove a man's lust 'through some herb or stone, or some occult natural means'.[17] Moreover, they explained that it was possible for witchcraft to stop bodies from approaching one another, to freeze a man's desire for intercourse, to disturb a man's imagination to make a woman appear loathsome, to prevent the erection of the penis, and to close off the seminary ducts to prevent the flow of seed and vital spirits to the privy parts.[18]

The devil's methods thus reflected the complete range of natural accidents that could interfere with the generative process. Early modern demonologists and writers on witchcraft retained medieval ideas about the devil's power. For this reason this chapter will consider both impotence magic and infertility magic. Although many treatises focused upon the inability of the husband to engage in sexual activity, which of course prevented conception, discussions about this issue also implicitly looked at the ability of witchcraft to interfere with the reproductive potential of both the male and female body and the ability to conceive. It is also worth noting that these two ideas were likely gendered: impotence magic in most cases was thought to affect only men, while magic that caused infertility, as will be seen, affected both the male and female body. Even though, superficially, these may have been seen as separate actions and problems, the texts examined here suggest that both problems, as when caused by a natural affliction, were viewed as inherently connected. Indeed, in *A dialogue of witches* (1575) Lambert Daneau wrote of the devil and his witches that

> they can hinder ye vertue & acte of generation, which is contayned w[ith]in ye bodie in certen vessels of seed, either by casting in by their venim an over coldnes of the vessels, or else raysing a certen hatred or misliking one of ye other betweene man & wife.[19]

---

[15] Richard Kieckhefer, *Magic in the Middle Ages*, Cambridge 2000, 9.
[16] Ibid.
[17] Heinrich Kramer and James Sprenger, *The Malleus maleficarum*, ed. and trans. Montague Summers, New York 1971, 55–6.
[18] Ibid. 55.
[19] Lambert Daneau, *A dialogue of witches in foretime named lot-tellers and now commonly called sorcerers*, London 1575, sig. 32r.

Daneau was clear here that it was both the fertility and sexual ability of the body that could be impeded; the devil could poison the body, perhaps with natural substances, or could make a man hate his wife and avoid having sex with her. Despite their chronological separation, both of these texts informed their readers that the devil could use natural and occult means to disrupt reproduction. This variety of methods reinforced the idea that the boundary between the natural and the preternatural was indeterminate. The *Malleus maleficarum* further emphasised this by explaining that the devil's greater knowledge allowed him to manipulate natural means in order to create occult effects:

> since the devil is more powerful than man, and man can obstruct the generative powers by means of frigid herbs ... much more can the devil do this, since he has greater knowledge and cunning.[20]

The *Malleus'* authors were clear that both men and the devil could damage the reproductive body. It was only the devil's greater knowledge and cunning that made him more adept at performing the operation. In many early modern treatises that addressed magical illness the authors often discussed causes that could be seen as either natural or preternatural. The use of herbs, stones and amulets to impose sterility was often described with little clarity about whether the effects were caused by magic, hidden virtues, or through the natural qualities of the object. The actions that Kramer and Sprenger described can be seen as the foundation upon and framework within which early modern opinions operated. These methods of procuring sterility were believed to be in use during the early modern period and were discussed by demonologists and medical authors alike.

Confusion surrounding the boundary between natural medical practice, which was legitimate in the period, and illicit witchcraft can clearly be identified in numerous seventeenth-century tracts. In his *Occult physick* (1660) William Williams, who styled himself '*Philosophus*' and '*Student in the Cœlistial Sciences*', aimed to present the magical and physical virtues of plants, beasts and herbs.[21] In the first book, which examines beasts, Williams listed various animal parts that could be used to cause impotence or barrenness. He wrote of the row-buck: 'Take the Horns of him and make Beads thereof, and wear them about your neck, or wrists, it causeth conception. And if a man weareth the same, he shall not have his natural course of Seed, though he lie with a woman.'[22] He provided no explanation of how the horns created these effects, but the title of the book implies that the physical virtues of the row-buck were passed into the body through proximity. Yet wearing beads

---

[20] Kramer and Sprenger, *Malleus maleficarum*, 55.
[21] William Williams, *Occult physic: or, The three principles in nature anatomized by a philosophical operation, taken from experience, in three books*, London 1660, title page.
[22] Ibid. 5. Williams also wrote (p. 3) of an amulet made of tortoise egg.

around the body was also reminiscent of amulets and charms worn upon the body to work effects through occult (hidden) means. It is interesting that the effects of these beads allowed for an erection which would mimic the shape of the phallic, and thus sexually stimulating, horn used while preventing conception. Yet horns, and the wearing of horns, were commonly used to represent a cuckold, a man whose wife has committed infidelity, because of her husband's inability to sexually satisfy her. Hence the horns simultaneously represented the erect and virile penis and impotence and cuckoldry in the man. What is clear in this example is that Williams did not provide his readers with a clear distinction between natural and magical. Tom Blaen has scrutinised the difficulties of this distinction and argued that stones and gemstones could easily be used for a range of legitimate medical or illicit purposes, which reflected pre-Reformation Church practices and aspects of popular piety.[23] The row-buck horn beads may have drawn upon legitimate religious, medical and occult elements that merely appeared superstitious following the Reformation. Once the legitimate sphere of their use had been removed the connotations of where these beads drew their power from could be reinterpreted by the reader as medical, occult or diabolical.

William Williams's text was a medical text and the occult virtues that he listed were not considered to be diabolical or dangerous. Similarly, *The magick of Kirani king of Persia and of Harpocration* (1685) discussed the magical and medicinal virtues of stones, herbs, fishes, beasts and birds without suggesting that these attributes were illicit.[24] This text, compiled between the fourth and the eighth centuries AD, had existed in the form of Latin translations since the twelfth and thirteenth centuries and was published in English in 1685.[25] The author stated that the '*Kirani* has many prodigious Virtues of things both in Medicine, and other Affairs' and the *Harpocration* is 'highly and deservedly valued by Learned Men'.[26] This work is extensive, containing remedies for a vast array of diseases, and the properties of numerous natural objects. Relatively few of these were imbued with the power to remove fertility, although the *Kiranides and Harpocration* included a two-part recipe to regulate conception, the first to ensure conception and the second so '*That she may not Conceive*'.[27] The contraceptive part of the recipe stated that 'if she have no mind to conceive let her gird her self with the ope[n] Seeds, [of the herb Peony], and the Wax of a Mules Ear; as lon[g] as she pleases'.[28] It

---

[23] Tom Blaen, 'The popular use of "precious" stones medicinally in early modern Scotland', in K. Georganta, F. Collignon and A.-M. Millim (eds), *The apothecary's chest: magic, art and medication*, Newcastle 2009, 83–95.

[24] Anon., *The magick of Kirani king of Persia; and of Harpocration; containing the magical and medicinal vertues of stones, herbs, fishes, beasts and birds*, London 1685.

[25] Catherine Rider, *Magic and impotence in the Middle Ages*, Oxford 2006, 23, 84.

[26] Anon., *The magick of Kirani*, sigs A4v–A5r.

[27] Ibid. 11–12.

[28] Ibid.

is likely that the open seeds were believed to have lost the generative virtue that would have been contained within them when sealed, while the mule is traditionally sterile. The recipe was presumably, therefore, designed to pass the sterile qualities of the seeds and the mule to the human body through proximity. However, this was only one part of the operation; in the first spell the ingredients were to be tied inside a linen cloth dyed seven different colours.[29] This suggests that the recipe performed some preternatural actions as seven was a number closely associated with magic. Accordingly this recipe also shows the indistinct boundary that existed between magical remedies and the natural actions of animals and plants.

The unclear distinction between the natural and occult properties of objects shows that the boundary between natural and preternatural causes of impotence inflicted from outside the body could be indistinct. The use of natural herbs and animal parts to cause sterility was often considered to be occult but natural, as can be seen in a variety of works.[30] The occult properties of plants, animal parts, or stones were given by God and, therefore, were a legitimate aspect of the natural world. As Kieckhefer has suggested, even though the idea of natural magic took a firm hold in European culture in the fourteenth and fifteenth centuries, it was not precisely defined; for many it merely referred to powers in nature that were not widely understood and aroused awe.[31] This lack of definition meant that even when herbs and stones were used for their natural properties it was still possible for their use to be reminiscent of spells and amulets associated with diabolism. The widespread acceptance of the indistinct boundary between the natural and the magical created a distinct setting in which medical writers could advocate the use of natural, sexually stimulating, remedies for the treatment of magically caused infertility.

In addition to the difficulties of distinguishing between magical and natural actions, early modern writers did not always delineate between the types of infertility caused by witchcraft or between the methods used to effect these results. William Drage's *Daimonomageia* (1665) stated in an all-encompassing manner that 'All Diseases that are caused by Nature, may be caused by Witchcraft; But all that are caused by Witchcraft, cannot be caused by nature', within which he included 'Barrenness ... Sterility and *Impotentia coeundi*' (impotence).[32] For an audience specifically interested in magical illness Drage, an apothecary and physician of Hitchin, Hertfordshire, demonstrated that different types of magic could cause different effects in the generative system. Although not a medical writer, Thomas

---

[29] Ibid.

[30] See Giambattista Della Porta, *Natural magick by John Baptista Porta, a Neopolitane: in twenty books*, London,1658, 17; Anon., *The magick of Kirani*, 17, 30.

[31] Kieckhefer, *Magic in the Middle Ages*, 12.

[32] William Drage, *Daimonomageia: a small treatise of sicknesses and diseases from witchcraft*, London 1665, 10.

Cooper also explained that witchcraft could cause a range of effects in the reproductive body that mirrored natural infertility; the devil could '*hinder the operations of nature*, and so may be a means to hinder copulation, and so procreation' by 'corrupting naturall heate', by making the penis inadequate for sexual activity, by making the seed too cold to be potent, by stealing away the seed entirely, or by making a man unable to have sex with his wife, even though he was still able to have sex with others.[33] Cooper provided his readers with detail about what magic could do to the reproductive organs, but provided no information about how victims could identify that their problems were a consequence of *maleficia*; he did not give a clear indication of the spells, enchantments or curses that would lead to these effects. This approach to discussing infertility magic was repeated by several medical writers who also did not distinguish the type or cause of magic that could result in infertility and impotence. For example, in the *Golden practice of physick* the authors explained that a '*Defect, or Want of Copulation*' could be caused 'also by inchantments, when the exquisite sense of the Yard is so lost that it will not rise by the tickling, which we shall shew proceedeth from the seed'.[34] Although the authors here were clear about what enchantments could do to the male genitalia they were not explicit about how these enchantments were enacted. The absence of this information in medical texts is not surprising given that cunning folk and illegitimate practitioners were often associated with ritualistic treatments and actions; medical writers were not inclined to include information of this sort even if they possessed it, in order to safeguard their reputations. The authors of this treatise stated, after another brief description of impotence magic, 'how this is done being preternatural, doth not concern us to enquire'.[35] Other medical texts were even more vague in their descriptions: the *Supreme mysteries of nature* by Paracelsus stated only that 'the loss of Strength and Virtue in the Members of Generation ... happens by divers accidents; some whereof are natural, others are against nature, by witchcraft'.[36] The language here stated that witchcraft was against nature. However, Stuart Clark has argued that all demonic activity was understood to happen within the laws of nature. Only God, through supernatural miracles, could work outside, or against, nature. Demonic magic worked entirely through natural powers; it only seemed to be against nature when compared to the powers of man.[37] There was no place in Christian theology and natural philosophy for the devil to exceed the limits of the natural world, as this would have challenged the funda-

---

[33] Thomas Cooper, *The mystery of witch-craft*, London 1617, 260–1.

[34] Platter, *A golden practice of physick*, 169.

[35] Ibid.

[36] Paracelsus, *Paracelsus of the supreme mysteries of nature ... translated by Robert Turner*, London 1655, 113.

[37] Stuart Clark, *Thinking with demons: the idea of witchcraft in early modern Europe*, Oxford 1997, 153.

mental order of the world.³⁸ Although this may broadly have been the case, this author's description would suggest that this interpretation of demonic activity was not universally understood.

Even though these discussions of infertility magic were rather vague, there were one or two types of witchcraft that were discussed frequently by theological and medical writers. The most commonly discussed method for causing impotence in a man was the ligature spell. However, the exact effects of the spell upon the generative organs were not necessarily recorded by early modern writers. In some cases it was not even made clear who the spell affected. Although often described as a male affliction, writers confusingly, discussed the spell in non-gendered terms. In 1597 James VI of Scotland published the *Dæmonologie* which stated that witches stopped 'maried folkes, to have naturallie adoe with [one] [an]other, (by knitting so manie knottes upon a poynt at the time of their marriage)'.³⁹ This passage neglected to inform the reader whether the man, woman or both would, be affected by this spell or which part of the act of generation was hindered. Similarly, Drage only provided a simple outline of the process of the ligature spell hinting that 'witches use certain words, which they mumble, and tie a knot',⁴⁰ although he did state that witches took away virility by preventing copulation or by preventing ejaculation.⁴¹ From these examples it is very difficult to establish how these spells intended to impede intercourse. It is possible that authors of texts such as these assumed that their readers would understand how these spells worked. Drage's statement also insinuated that there were different ways in which these spells could operate, either preventing intercourse or preventing conception. The incomprehensibility of these spells exists in stark contrast to the explicit physical explanations of reproductive failure found in the medical literature. Subsequently this may have caused medical writers, practitioners and victims to resort to a natural, understandable, means of treatment such as sexual stimulants.

Even in cases where the author was clear about the gender of the intended victim the actions of the spell were not always apparent. This is not surprising given that magic was partly identifiable by its incomprehensibility. Moreover, to spread clear information about these spells was to demystify them, removing some of their power. Francis Bacon, in his philosophical work *Sylva sylvarum* (1627), described how

> In *Zant*, it is very ordinary, to make *Men Impotent*, to accompany with their *Wives*. The like is Practised in *Gasconie*; Where it is called *Nouër l'eguilltte*. It is practiced always upon the *Wedding Day*. And in *Zant*, the Mothers

---

[38] Ibid. 168.
[39] James VI, king of Scotland, *Daemonologie, in forme of a dialogue, divided into three books*, Edinburgh 1597, 12.
[40] Drage, *Daimonomageia*, 14.
[41] Ibid.

themselves doe it, by way of Prevention; Because thereby they hinder other *Charmes*, and can undoe their Owne.[42]

Although Bacon declared that this spell was used to make men impotent this label was applied to a range of sexual and reproductive failures in the male body. Hence it is not clear whether the man's sexual desire had been dampened or whether he was unable to have and maintain an erection. Bacon described the ligature spell as a form of preventative enchantment to repel the charms, most likely impotence or seduction spells, of other women. In this instance, the mother took action on the day of the wedding and then removed the charm for the wedding night, allowing the conjugal duties to take place, legitimising the marriage. When used in this way the ligature spell rather counter-intuitively acted as a way of ensuring copulation.

All of these descriptions of the ligature spell were rather vague, from a modern perspective. It is likely that most men and women understood it as a form of natural magic, the manipulation of the occult (hidden) properties of the natural world to create a particular effect. However the actions and effects of the spell would also have resonated with broader cultural ideas of the period. One possible interpretation of the spell was that it mimicked the action of actually tying a ligature around the penis, preventing the necessary emission of seminal fluid. The ligature may also have reflected ideas about marriage and the family. In the *Preparative to marriage* (1591) Henrie Smith stated that 'Marriage is called *Conjugium*, which signifieth a knitting or joining together.'[43] From this it could be inferred that marriage 'knits' two people together and so restricts the number of sexual partners. This restriction was perhaps reflected in the ligature spell where the outcome was specifically intended to prevent a man having sexual relations with his wife, or a particular woman. Beyond these specific possible interpretations, it is also plausible that that 'tying', 'knitting' and 'knots' were all simply suggestive of binding, twisting and tangling, which thus symbolised a restriction of generative power, perhaps more specifically the seminal vessels: the 1664 edition of Felix Platter's *Golden practice of physick* suggested that this incantation left men bound 'because it is caused by tying of a Point, a Bulls pizle, or Wolfes pizle, or of some other Lecherous beast'.[44] In this case the mirroring of physically tying the genitalia was clear.

The magick of Kirani king of Persia provided its readers with a very detailed description of the ligature spell and its effects, which appears in stark contrast to the previous examples. Like James VI, the author believed that the spell could affect both men and women. The book included instructions on how to create and conduct the spell:

---

[42] Bacon, *Sylva sylvarum*, 235–6.
[43] Henrie Smith, *A preparative to marriage*, London 1591, 56.
[44] Felix Platter, *Platerus golden practice of physic*, London 1664, 169.

Upon the Stone *Opsarius* engrave a Man having his Privities cut off, placed or lying at his Feet, and his hands contracted underneath; and himself reaching down to his Privities, and behind his back let there be *Venus*, having back to back, she turning herself, and seeing him. Enclose therefore the Stone of the Fish *Cynædius*. But if you have not one of them which are under the head, you must put underneath the Root of the Herb, and the end of the Bird's left wing. Enclose it in a large Gold Box, and you must put it into a thong of the nerve of a Hawk's Stomach, let it be thin, sewing it in the middle of the thong or nerve, that it do not appear. This is that which is painted in the head of *Venus*, comprehended in the thong or ligature, which is called *Cestus*. *That a Male may not erect*; If any one touch a Male with the thong or ligature, he will not erect, and if he carries it unknowingly he grows effeminate ... And if a Woman carry this ligature, none will carnally lie with her. For the Man cannot erect.[45]

The spell was not intended to affect the female body directly or render women infertile. Instead it was, again, the man's sexual performance that was debilitated. This reflected the descriptions from the *Malleus maleficarum* and other texts where it was believed that diabolical magic could prevent a man from approaching a woman. The relative consistency with which these spells were described as affecting the male body is potentially significant: the affliction of the male body, which was seen as more likely to be sexually potent and functional than the female body, by external forces conceivably induced shame. The man was not able to please the woman in any way, could not pay her due benevolence, and he could not get her with child. Similarly ligature spells of this nature, which created a specific physical effect in the male body, represented a form of transgression: the witch obtained power and control over the male form. It may have been, therefore, that relatively few cases of the ligature spell were reported because men who believed that they had been affected by such as spell did not want to admit that they had lost control over their own physicality and sexuality.

In addition to the ligature spell, authors often described many methods for imposing barrenness and impotence that could be classed as enchantments.[46] Enchantments involved the use of rituals and symbols to communicate with demons and spirits in order to enact particular desires and effects. Often this involved placing an object within the victim's house or in close proximity to his/her body. These spells were thought to affect individuals, couples or

---

[45] Anon., *The magick of Kirani*, 32–3. The stone Opsarius may be the stone taken from a type of Asian fish. However the term is not found in the OED. Cestus was a girdle worn by brides or a girdle associated specifically with Venus: OED, s.v. 'cestus', accessed 23 June 2013.

[46] It was also believed that witches could cast a 'glamour' over the penis, which removed the organ or all sensory perception of it. This was rarely mentioned in medical texts: Reginald Scot, *Scot's Discovery of witchcraft*, London [1584] 1651, 60–1. See also Stephens, 'Witches who steal penises', 495–516, and *Demon lovers: witchcraft, sex and the crisis of belief*, Chicago–London 2002; and Cameron, *Enchanted Europe*, 35.

whole households. Drage described one of these methods in *Daimonomageia* (1665):

> A Woman of *Onipontus*, wonderfully tortured, was freed by taking away a waxen Image an hands length, laid under the threshold of the door by a Witch; the Image was bored through, and two pins stuck in each side, which so tormented this woman. Another laid a beast like a Toad, under the threshold of a door, and made Barrenness to all the house.[47]

In this case a waxen image and a toad were laid under the threshold of the house. The waxen image was used in both ancient Greek erotic spells and curses and medieval necromancy.[48] The toad-like beast could also have been imbued with the power to remove fertility; it is likely that the toad was thought to be the witch's familiar, able to harm victims according to the witch's desire.[49] Both Drage and R. B., the author of *The kingdom of darkness* (1688), described a man who was made impotent when a witch placed an earthenware pot full of enchantments in the well inside his courtyard.[50] This, presumably, allowed the spell to affect numerous members of the household. As with the toad, this spell brought reproductive failure to multiple victims, the nobleman and his new wife. Once again the ways in which this spell affected the couple are not made clear; the couple's ability to engage in intercourse may have been hindered, or their ability to conceive could have been damaged. Understanding the process or specific effects of the enchantment was not considered crucial to identifying the magic or removing it. Although it may appear from these texts that the authors were credulous about magic, Bernard Capp has emphasised that Drage's treatise was mainly concerned with finding treatments for diseases caused by witchcraft, not

---

[47] Drage, *Daimonomageia*, 14; ODNB, s.v. 'William Drage', accessed 23 June 2013.

[48] Christopher Faraone, *Ancient Greek love magic*, Cambridge, MA 2001; Derek Collins, *Magic in the ancient Greek world*, Oxford 2008, 88–104; Richard Kieckhefer, 'Necromancy', in William W. Kibler and Grover A. Zinn (eds), *Medieval France: an encyclopaedia*, New York–London 1995, 661–2, and *Magic in the Middle Ages*, 60, 82–3; Bengt Ankarloo, Stuart Clark and William Monter, *Witchcraft and magic in Europe: the period of the witch trials*, London 2002, 82.

[49] Several texts mention the use of toads as familiars: Scot, *Scot's Discovery of witchcraft*, 147; Anon., *The apprehension and confession of three notorious witches*, London 1589, sig. Br. See also James Sharpe, *Instruments of darkness: witchcraft in England, 1550–1750*, London 1996, 71, and Barbara Rosen, *Witchcraft in England, 1558–1618*, Amherst 1991, pp. xi, 47–8, 71, 110, 115, 160.

[50] R. B., *The kingdom of darkness: or, The history of daemons, spectres, witches, apparitions, possessions, disturbances, and other wonderful and supernatural delusions, mischievious feats, and malicious impostures of the devil*, London 1688, 93. R. B. recorded that 'an earthen pot filled with inchantments … of which the old woman [witch] did affirm, that as long as it lay there you should both be disabled as to generation'. See also Drage, *Daimonomageia*, 14. Drage included this type of magic in his section on taking 'away virility, and that a man and wife should not copulate'. He noted that 'One was so bound by an earthen Pot, threw by a Witch into his Well, with some Ceremonies'.

with identifying and punishing witches.[51] Thus, even when describing cases of infertility magic authors such as Drage were keen to retain and advocate a naturalistic response.

The use of these enchantments within the house or close to the body drew upon older ideas of sympathetic magic. Euan Cameron has noted that by the late Middle Ages it was conventional to accept that a bent needle, which represented failed erection, placed in a man's bed would cause impotence.[52] A similar idea was also discussed by John of Gaddesden. In his *Rosa anglica* (c. 1320), he related that 'a needle with which a dead man has been sewn up, fixed in the bed or in a man or woman's clothes when they should have intercourse, impedes the erection of the penis and consequently generation' which he took from the eighth book of Constantine's *Practica*.[53] A spell from *The magick of King Kirani* (1685) used a similar method, recommending that vervain should be laid under the pillow of the victim, bewitching the marital bed, or the specific place in which intercourse was likely to happen.[54] It is apparent then that early modern enchantments followed these older examples quite closely. Nevertheless, it is uncertain whether scholars and laymen understood exactly how these spells worked. For many readers it was accepted that only the Devil was privy to this knowledge. To print details of how these spells worked demystified them and made them accessible to anyone. Hence it was often cases of infertility and impotence deemed to be inexplicable that were considered to be the result of witchcraft.

The discussions of infertility magic found in a range of witchcraft and medical treatises show that, even when not always fully explained, medical writers and the wider populace acknowledged that there was a variety of ways in which infertility spells could be enacted. It was also accepted that infertility magic could cause a range of effects in the reproductive organs; as the *Malleus* explained, the devil could affect the amount of desire and pleasure felt by the victim, prevent the movement of seminal fluid, impede erection and make the woman appear loathsome.[55] The Devil thus had the power to prevent sexual intercourse altogether or allow it to happen in a fruitless state where no offspring would be produced. Each of these results echoed natural causes of impotence and barrenness. Consequently, medical

---

[51] ODNB, s.v. 'William Drage', accessed 23 June 2013.
[52] Cameron, *Enchanted Europe*, 35.
[53] Cited in Rider, *Magic and impotence*, 168.
[54] Anon., *The magick of Kirani*, 30.
[55] R. B., *The kingdom of darkness*, 92. The author includes the story of a man who by embracing the object of his desire caused her to die. This story reflected the idea that the devil could manipulate feelings of love and desire and the idea that he could physically prevent intercourse. It is apparent that the *Malleus* was still being read in the seventeenth century as it is mentioned in several treatises, for example John Cotta, *The triall of witch-craft*, London 1616, 58, 90, and Anon., *A pleasant treatise of witches their imps, and meetings*, London 1673, 3.

writers believed and advocated to their readers that it was possible to treat and cure magical infertility with natural remedies, and in particular with aphrodisiacs.

Scepticism and decline

The acceptance of magically induced infertility was not, however, consistent across the early modern period. Increasingly in the seventeenth and eighteenth centuries authors were sceptical about witchcraft. Reginald Scot, a sixteenth-century writer on witchcraft, emphatically denounced the reputation of witches in his *Discovery of witchcraft* (1584). Despite his desire to prove that witches were *'imaginary Erroneous conceptions and novelties'*, Scot's text still presented information on witchcraft to his readers and thus may have helped to perpetuate belief in witchcraft and magic.[56] Indeed he was cited in many subsequent treatises on witchcraft, many of which attacked his scepticism.[57] He, for example, presented information on the actions of witches reproduced directly from prior texts, such as the *Malleus maleficarum*.[58] Scot suggested that belief in *maleficium* was widespread. He argued that people 'affirme, that the vertue of generation is impeached by witches, both inwardly, and outwardly: for intrinsecally [sic] they repress the courage, and they stop the passage of the mans seed, so as it may no[t] descend to the vessels of generation'.[59] Scot's confidence that these beliefs were widespread in England, however, is not substantiated by recorded cases of infertility magic, which are few.[60] Although treatises extolled that the devil and his witches could cause infertility, few were willing to state that they had been affected in this way. It is plausible that this reflected a desire to hide afflictions of this nature; procreation was a natural bodily function ordained by God, to lose control over which might therefore have been particularly shameful. Moreover, the fact that it was most likely a female witch who disrupted a man's control over his body may have fed into patriarchal concerns about male authority and leadership. Hence, for men in particular, this form of impotence may have been deeply shaming making sufferers less inclined to publicise or record their problems. Alternatively, as has been shown, infertility witchcraft and magic was thought to manifest in

---

[56] Scot, *Scot's Discovery of witchcraft*, title page; S. F. Davies, 'The reception of Reginald Scot's *Discovery of witchcraft*: witchcraft, magic, and radical religion', *JHI* lxxiv/3 (2013), 381–401 at p. 393.

[57] Davies, 'The reception of Reginald Scot', 383.

[58] Ibid. Scot noted that his information, including some on reproduction and sexuality, came from the *Malleus maleficarum*, 7, 59, 60.

[59] Scot, *Scot's Discovery of witchcraft*, 60.

[60] I am grateful to Dr Marion Gibson who confirmed that this type of magic was rare and that the two cases I have encountered may have been the only ones recorded in England.

ways that were inherently related to natural bodily problems. It may simply have been that many patients readily accepted that their failure to conceive was a natural problem rather than ascribing their difficulties to witchcraft. Given the lack of recorded discussion about this issue it is difficult to establish definitively how people thought about, or responded to, witchcraft and infertility magic.

Several medical writers also demonstrated scepticism about the ability of witches to cause impotence and infertility. Some medical writers like William Salmon merely stated that 'as for Authors talk of the Stars and Enchantments, I have ever been dubious in the Case'.[61] A few practitioners not only noted that they did not believe in witchcraft, but argued that it was only the young, and gullible, who believed that *maleficia* was the cause of their reproductive problems: a late seventeenth-century translation of the works of Michael Ettmüller disdainfully explained that 'we have several Instances in new married Youngsters, that fancy themselves bewitch'd'.[62] Similarly Mattheus Purmann's anecdote about witchcraft involved a victim who was twenty-eight years old, newly married and 'tormented with the apprehension that his Wife had bewitched him, and would not be perswaded [sic] to the contrary, by all the Arguments we could use against so Foolish an Opinion'.[63] These authors were clear that it was folly to believe in this type of magic and suggested that beliefs of this kind were a source of frustration when they interfered with natural treatment regimes.

Throughout the eighteenth century scepticism about the powers and reality of witchcraft increased. This was reflected in a substantial reduction in the publication of texts that dealt with this topic as a physical reality. Those works that did discuss witchcraft increasingly pointed out that there was little question about the reality of witchcraft: it was merely illusion employed to deceive ignorant and gullible members of the populace. As those who have previously examined witchcraft in the eighteenth century have observed, the attitudes of the educated at this time were mostly ambivalent.[64] Many people believed that witchcraft had ceased to exist in their own era, but did not reject the idea that it was possible or had occurred previously.[65]

One reason for the decline in the acceptance of witchcraft was the rise, across the seventeenth century, of Cartesian rationalism. This complex epistemological change, which reassessed the relationship between the mind and the body, brought about a reinterpretation of the ability of spirits and devils to

---

[61] Salmon, *Systema medicinale*, 240.
[62] Ettmüller, *Etmullerus abridg'd*, 573.
[63] Purmannus, *Chirurgia curiosa*, 144.
[64] Owen Davies, *Witchcraft, magic and culture, 1736–1951*, Manchester–New York 1999, 7–16; Ian Bostridge, *Witchcraft and its transformation, c. 1650–1750*, Oxford 1997, ch. v.
[65] Davies, *Witchcraft, magic and culture*, 8.

influence the natural world. Cartesianism's separation of the physical and the mental realms only allowed for God and man as causal agencies in the world.[66] By prioritising the agency of God, Cartesian philosophy had the potential to relegate devils and spirits from the natural world. Thus, with its introduction and interpretation, scholars were able to disavow the power of the devil to interfere with the corporeal human body.[67] The rejection of witchcraft, however, was not merely the result of one factor but involved the interplay of social, religious and political elements. As Owen Davies has demonstrated, witchcraft debates became fused with political and religious disagreements. Tories, conservative in both their political and religious beliefs, continued to follow the literal truth of the Bible and so maintained a belief in witchcraft, while progressive, free-thinking Whigs became associated with scepticism and witchcraft denial.[68] Not only did the involvement of politics change attitudes to witchcraft, it also suppressed vociferous discussions of the topic.[69]

Some authors did still discuss witchcraft, albeit briefly. Robert Johnson's *Praxis medicinae reformata* (1700) only noted that 'Some are of the opinion that Witch-craft may be the cause [of barrenness].'[70] Johnson not only failed to provide any detail about magic of this kind but also distanced himself from those who believed in such things. Texts that discussed witchcraft at length, from a medical perspective, were much rarer. One example was Richard Boulton's *Compleat history of magick, sorcery, and witchcraft* (1715). Boulton was a medical writer who had earlier published works on muscular motion and the heat of the blood.[71] Yet, even in this case, witchcraft was not scrutinised with the same levels of concern as in the seventeenth century. Moreover, although Boulton gave credence to the contemporary presence of witches, stating that 'the Being of Witches is undeniable', he was not inclined to accept infertility enchantment in the same way.[72] He described how there were spells that caused lust and hatred, and stated that some practised magic by tying knots, but he did not relate these practices to infertility or impotence.[73] Boulton's treatise was perhaps a good indicator of the ideas of the wider contemporary populace: Ian Bostridge has described it as a familiar collection of narratives lacking any detailed analytical

---

[66] J. A. van Ruler, 'Minds, forms, and spirits: the nature of Cartesian disenchantment', *JHI* lxi/3 (2000), 381–95 at p. 387.
[67] Ibid. 383, 384, 391.
[68] Davies, *Witchcraft, magic and culture*, 8–9.
[69] Ibid. 9.
[70] Johnson, *Praxis medicinae reformata*, 246.
[71] *ODNB*, s.v. 'Richard Boulton', accessed 20 June 2013.
[72] Richard Boulton, *A compleat history of magick, sorcery and witchcraft*, London 1715–16, 11. Boulton described (pp. 7–17) the actions that the devil could teach his followers, but made no mention of impotence magic.
[73] Ibid. 7–17, 175.

work.[74] He has also argued that the *History of magick* was an anachronism, trying to participate in a debate that had been denied much of its theological grounding.[75] Later eighteenth-century works also dismissed Boulton's views as weak and beneath contempt.[76] Thus it is evident that educated scholars in the eighteenth-century found continued belief in all of aspects witchcraft contemptible, not just infertility bewitchment.

Other eighteenth-century authors treated the sexual components of witchcraft with comparable disregard. The anonymous text, *A discourse on witchcraft* (1736), reproached the folly of men for allowing the belief that witches could destroy 'the Fruit of the Womb, at their Pleasure' or 'enable and disable in Matters venereal'.[77] By 1736 this derision was not uncommon. This was the year in which the Witchcraft Statute removed the reality of the witch from the law: all those who pretended to use enchantments or sorcery were to be subject to punishment.[78] In both literature and law, the reality of the witch was eradicated and condemned as a historical *persona* no longer relevant to contemporary culture. The trend for criticising earlier beliefs about infertility bewitchment developed further in later eighteenth-century texts which simply neglected to discuss this form of magic. *The compleat wizzard*, published in 1770, failed to mention impotence enchantments or the ability of witches to impede conception.[79] This absence was perhaps the culmination of a selective and progressive move away from the sexualised elements of witchcraft belief. For a number of authors it was no longer reasonable to give credence to these particular elements. This shift may simply have reflected the broader changes in witchcraft belief and law that were occurring across the eighteenth century. However, the rarity of witchcraft cases of this nature in England likely contributed to their rapid dismissal by scholars and medical writers.

Treating magically-induced infertility and impotence

For those who believed themselves to be bewitched there were three main means of treatment: prayer and fasting; using occult and ritualistic means to

---

[74] Bostridge, *Witchcraft and its transformation*, 139.
[75] Ibid. 141.
[76] Ibid. 142.
[77] Anon., *A discourse on witchcraft: occasioned by a bill now depending in parliament*, London 1736, 15.
[78] Davies, *Witchcraft, magic and culture*, 2.
[79] Anon., *The compleat wizzard ... together with several wonderful instances of the effects of witchcraft*, London 1770, 272–4. This tract still allowed for the idea that magic could be used in relation to love and desire; it recited spells which allowed a woman to see her future husband. Similarly Boulton's earlier work allowed that the devil could bend the minds and wills of men towards 'extraordinary and unreasonable Desires and Lusts': *A compleat history of magick*, 174.

remove the spell potentially employing the help of a cunning man or wise woman; or following medical and theological advice and employing natural remedies, such as aphrodisiacs. In this way sexual stimulants were, again, employed to restore the generative capabilities of the body. The evidence presented here must be treated with caution. Discussions about the treatment of infertility witchcraft were rare in early modern printed works. It was a subject often couched in scepticism, criticism and derision. Medical authors viewed illness induced by witchcraft with a degree of cynicism and therefore failed to debate the subject in printed works. Printing material of this nature was also thought to demystify the occult process and thereby popularise and democratise it. Consequently authors wishing to protect the status and power of magical rites and rituals did not write and print explanations of magic and magical healing. The absence of this evidence appears in stark contrast to the frequent and lengthy descriptions of natural sexual stimulants seen in medical treatises. Accordingly, the argument portrayed here draws together oddments and brief comments from disparate genres which only provide oblique access to the topic. Thus, although this section discusses the entire period between 1550 and 1780, it is difficult to argue definitively that a cohesive or unified appreciation of the remedies was ever achieved or disseminated. Nonetheless, the sources that do discuss this issue strongly suggest that a natural response, using aphrodisiac treatments, was central to medical practitioners' responses to cases where patients felt that they had been bewitched.

Non-medical texts from across the period did describe various rituals or actions that would remove an enchantment or curse. In order to unveil their stupidity, Reginald Scot's *Discovery of witchcraft* listed 'Certain popish and magicall cures, for them that are bewitched in their privities.'[80] Scot's tract provided a means to express his virulent oppositions to Catholicism.[81] Amongst the many elements of the Catholic faith that Scot opposed was the use of medicinal prayers and charms.[82] In particular, Scot wanted people to resist the temptation to inscribe the divine, supernatural or miraculous to natural occurrences just because they were beyond comprehension.[83] In this section of his work Scot described several ritualistic remedies for infertility magic that likely would have been considered superstitious by many Protestants. Although the ways in which these remedies acted was not explicitly described, they may have functioned on the edge of or outside of the medical framework. A popular cure was to 'pisse through a wedding ring'; another required the 'smoak of the tooth of a dead man'; while another required the

---

[80] Scot, *Scot's Discovery of witchcraft*, 63.
[81] Leland L. Estes, 'Reginald Scot and his *Discoverie of witchcraft*: religion and science in the opposition to the European witch craze', *Church History* lii/4 (1983), 444–56 at p. 446.
[82] Ibid.
[83] Ibid. 451.

victim to 'fill a quill with quick-silver, and lay the same under the cushin, where such a one sitteth, or else to put it under the threshold of the door of the house or chamber where he dwelleth'.[84] These remedies demonstrate a rather eclectic collection of ideas. The quill filled with quick-silver follows the means by which these enchantments could be enacted, perhaps functioning as a form of counter magic. Conversely the 'smoak' of the tooth of a dead man would appear, from its lack of accompanying explanation, to function through occult, or hidden, means to remove the impediment upon the genitals. The last two measures that Scot listed were variations on traditional church practices: 'when ones instrument of venery is bewitched, certain characters must be written [o]n virgin-parchment, celebrated and holyed by a popish priest and thereon also must the 141. Psalme be written, and bound *ad viri fascinati coxam*'.[85] The final remedy required a waxen image of the bewitched member to be offered at St Anthony's altar, to be sanctified by the mass.[86] Both of these were corruptions of existing church practices, intercession and the mass. Through this disparagement Scot was able to state that 'popish' cures were equivalent to superstitious magical practices. He listed this varied group of remedies and actions together to highlight that all measures of combating impotence of this kind were irregular. Scot's underlying theological assumptions, however, were not widely accepted, and it may have been that his sceptical remarks were disregarded by the majority of his readers.[87] Although Scot was representative in terms of his anti-popish views, he does not necessarily provide a representative account of early modern beliefs about witchcraft. Despite Scot's scorn for these 'cures' and his explicit identification of them with the Catholic Church, his work emphasises that when faced with infertility witchcraft, people had an assortment of popular measures at their disposal.

Some medical writers included remedies for infertility magic that could be viewed as forms of counter-magic or means to ward off witchcraft. For example Nicholas Culpeper's translation of Lazarus Riverius' *Practice of physick* explained that if barrenness had been caused by witchcraft then there was 'little place for Physick' because prayers and supplications to the Almighty were the appropriate means for gaining a cure.[88] However, he also noted that there were some methods by which a person could protect themselves from infertility magic:

> certaine Amulets are propounded by Authors, which have a peculiar vertue to resist the malignity of such Medicaments. *Cardan* will have it, that the Pizzle of a Wolf worn about the woman, will frustrate all such Incantations and

---

[84] Scot, *Scot's Discovery of witchcraft*, 64.
[85] Ibid. Approximate translation is 'for a man bewitched in the hip'.
[86] Ibid.
[87] Estes, 'Reginald Scot and his *Discoverie of witchcraft*', 455.
[88] Riverius, *The practice of physick* (1655 edn), 506.

fascinations. Others do much commend the Adamant and Hyacinth Stone. The Antients called Saint John-wort, the Divel-driver. The same vertue is likewise attributed to the Squil or Sea-Onion, to Eryngus, sagapenum, Rue, & other things, being worn by Man & Wife. Also certain it is, that for the parties concerned, to endeavour confidently to despise and slight all Charmes and Witch-crafts, is very profitable in this case. Also (if the Author of the Witch-craft be not known) it is good for them to Change their Habitation, and to forsake their Houses, Beds, wearing Cloathes, and other Houshold stuff, wherein the Charmes are oftentimes concealed.[89]

Similarly, in 1700, Robert Johnson wrote that 'If it be caused by Witch-craft, there are some things commended by Authours to be worn about the party against Fascination, *viz.* the Pizle of a Wolf, a Diamond, a Jacinth-stone, Rue, Squills, Sea-holly, *Sagapenum, Amara dulcis, Hypericon,* &c.'[90] It should be noted, however, that sea holly and the pizzle (penis) of a wolf were also thought to be aphrodisiacs. Substances like this blurred the boundaries between remedies designed to prevent infertility magic being enacted and those that restored and reinvigorated the reproductive organs, curing them of infertility.

Some ritualistic remedies that were designed not to prevent *maleficia* but to remove and reverse the effects of a spell or enchantment were also described by medical writers. In his 1684 treatise *Mercurius compitalitius* the Swiss physician Theophile Bonet informed his readers of numerous remedies for impotence, both of natural and preternatural origins. He claimed that the following remedy was useful for those who were bewitched: 'Take the Patient's Urine, as much as you please, boyl it in a pot covered, and if anyone have bewitched him, he that did it will be in great anxiety, will discover himself, and take off the Inchantment.'[91] This bears a resemblance to the drawing of a witch's blood to end an enchantment. By taking such an action the patient intended to force the witch to remove the spell or for the magic to be turned back upon them, consequently returning the generative body to its natural state. Some practitioners also used amulets or charms to appease popular understandings of witchcraft. John Webster, a physician and surgeon practising in Clitheroe, suggested that physicians should foster patients' fantasies in order to treat them.[92] While describing the treatment of melancholy patients by rational physicians he argued that 'if you should by plain reasons shew them, that they are decievied, and that there is no such matter, but that it is a natural disease, say what you can they shall not believe

---

[89] Ibid. 506–7. See also Sharp, *The midwives book*, 101, and Anon., *The English midwife enlarged*, 178.
[90] Johnson, *Praxis medicinae*, 248.
[91] Bonet, *Mercurius compitalitius*, 546.
[92] Cited in Lindsey Fitzharris, 'Magic, mysticism and medicine: the medical career of John Webster', in Georganta, Collignon and Millim, *The apothecary's chest*, 19–128 at p. 125.

you, but account you a Physician of small or no value'.[93] Thus, he concluded, physicians should 'indulge their fancy and seem to concur in opinion with them, and hang any insignificant thing about their necks, assuring them that it is a most efficacious and powerful charm, you may then easily settle their imaginations, and then give them that which is proper to eradicate the cause of their disease'.[94] Although Webster appears to be unique in arguing that ritualistic remedies were suitable in this way, his work does imply that the use of ritualistic remedies was driven by patients rather than practitioners. However, it is possible that many patients did accept the advice of their medical practitioners and followed a course of physick and regimen in order to treat infertility that they believed to have been caused by magic.

Commentary on infertility witchcraft was uncommon in the eighteenth century. In an exceptional and rare extract from the *New practice of physick* (1753) Peter Shaw noted that in cases of sterility, where neither party appeared to be at fault and thus witchcraft was thought to be the cause, 'amulets, charms, and magic rites are prescribed for the cure'.[95] Despite the rapid decline, in the eighteenth century, of medical discussion surrounding witchcraft of this kind, Shaw related this information without scepticism or criticism. Even so, his intention could have been to highlight that these remedies were a lingering remnant of previous practice. Although Shaw stated that these remedies were 'prescribed' it is not clear who was prescribing their use and he may have been referring to the practices of cunning men, wise women and quacks, rather than legitimate medical practitioners. Keith Thomas has suggested that many men and women turned to the remedies and rituals offered by cunning folk after the Reformation, which had effectively removed the wealth of healing resources offered by the pre-Reformation Church.[96] Shaw's statement does imply some measure of continued practice; however, the unified response of medical practitioners to this issue conversely implies that many men and women used natural remedies prescribed by medical practitioners to cure infertility magic. Thus, it is perhaps more accurate to argue that early modern men and women employed a dual strategy, which incorporated 'superstitious' rituals and natural medications in order to cure this affliction.

Most medical authors and church authorities advised patients who believed that they were the victims of witchcraft to pray to God for a cure and adopt natural humoural treatments. As has been shown, the level of scepticism relating to the power of witchcraft, particularly its ability to impede the genitals, was growing across the early modern period. Stuart Clark has also

---

[93] John Webster, *The displaying of supposed witchcraft*, London 1677, 323.

[94] Ibid. 324. For a discussion of the French context see Petry, 'Many such things surpass our knowledge', 55.

[95] Peter Shaw, *A new practice of physick: wherein the various disease incident to the human body are described*, London 1753, 458–9.

[96] Thomas, *Religion and the decline of magic*, 209–23.

shown that early modern scholars almost unanimously agreed that the devil and witches could only act according to the laws of nature.[97] In cases where witchcraft was acknowledged as the cause of a person's sexual and reproductive incapacity, it was understood that this impediment was produced naturally, within the boundaries of the natural world, and thus could be cured with natural herbs and foodstuffs, such as provokers of lust. This is reflected in the derogatory tone which Scot used in listing these 'popish' and 'magicall' cures. It was also revealed in the attitude of the Church to the Frances Howard case. The trial of Frances Howard took place in 1613 and a published version of the proceedings was produced from the papers of Francis Bacon in 1651. Parts of these papers may have been published previously and it is possible that this later retelling of the events of the trial does not contain an accurate portrayal of the Church's attitudes at the time. Nonetheless, in this version of the narrative, the archbishop of Canterbury, George Abbott, noted that there were only two legitimate courses of action to be taken in this situation: he stated that 'if there should be any, which should seem to be molested, we are taught to use two remedies, the one spiritual physick, the other external'.[98] The spiritual physic he referred to was fasting and prayer.[99] The external physic recommended was 'corporal medicine to be applyed there with, as against a disease'.[100] In this case the Church and theology supported the medical paradigm of treating infertility witchcraft with the appropriate natural remedies. Medical writers like Lazarus Riverius advocated a response based upon prayer and supplication to God for a cure. Similarly Jane Sharp, who noted that witchcraft could be the cause of infertility, wrote, of all types of barrenness, that 'Prayer is then the chief remedy of their barrenness, not neglecting such natural means, to further conception and to remove impediments that *God* hath appointed.'[101]

The endorsement of 'physick' as the appropriate treatment for impotence and infertility enchantments was not unique to the early modern period but, like demonological discussions, drew upon examples from the medieval period. For example, John of Gaddesden wrote in the *Rosa anglica* (1320), while discussing sterility, that a confection made of figs, nuts, hazelnuts, almonds and ginger was good even against poisons and *maleficia*.[102] This remedy contained many well-known aphrodisiacs and was evidently supposed to sexually stimulate the body. Catherine Rider has shown that medieval medical writers offered treatments to bewitched patients which

---

[97] Clark, *Thinking with demons*, 152.
[98] Francis Bacon, *A true and historical relation of the poysoning of Sir Thomas Overbury ... also, all the passages concerning the divorce between Robert, late earle of Essex, and the Lady Frances Howard*, London 1651, 5; ODNB, s.v. 'George Abbot', accessed 9 Aug. 2013.
[99] Bacon, *A true and historical relation*, 6.
[100] Ibid.
[101] Sharp, *The midwives book*, 178.
[102] Cited in Rider, *Magic and impotence in the Middle Ages*, 168.

had specifically aphrodisiac qualities: they were accompanied by descriptions such as, 'it powerfully excites intercourse', 'they excite the generative force marvellously' and 'it makes a great erection of the penis'.[103] These were not attributed with any occult virtues and, Rider stated, they appeared 'with no suggestion that there was anything magical involved in the original impotence'.[104] This approach again fits with Clark's argument that the limitations of diabolical power were well established.[105] It was widely acknowledged that God had provided man with the remedies necessary to combat diseases and disorders and that these were found in the bounty of the natural world. Medical writers consequently focused on the body itself when treating magically induced infertility and impotence using natural remedies not to remove the spell or enchantment but to rectify the effects of the magic. Jakob Rueff amalgamated his recipes for natural and preternatural sterility, drawing no distinction between the forms of treatment needed. He noted only that 'It remaineth also to speak a few words of those things which are to be ministred inwardly. For because the fruitfulnesse of man and wife may be hindred very much for want of desire to be acquainted with Venus ... disability of ingendering and effecting Conception ... or by the inchantments of evil arts.'[106] Here Rueff underlined the inextricable link between the pleasurable stimulation of the body and the ability to conceive, and connected these factors to the effects of witchcraft. Thus, he implicitly suggested that there was no difference in the treatment required. By using provokers of venery, which were believed to increase the desire and pleasure of the body, the effects of *maleficia* on the genitals could be overcome. Later in the period the authors of a *Golden practice of physick* adopted a similar position: although they acknowledged witchcraft as a cause of impotence and infertility they did not advocate any ritualistic cures. Instead they listed numerous remedies for a '*want of Copulation*' that were applicable no matter the cause of the problem. Only at the end of this section was it explained that 'Other things belong to the Cure of Incantations, as shaking of Pillows, pissing through the wedding-ring, or the Axle-tree of the Plough, or the changing of shifts, before they go to the sport, shiftings of the left foot, and the likes, these belong not to us. Nor care we for Amulets.'[107] The authors were categorical that these were not cures that would be used by a physician. More important, they offered no suggestion that these remedies would work, implying that victims/patients would be better served by using the many aphrodisiacs described on the preceding pages.

---

[103] Ibid. 173.
[104] Ibid.
[105] Clark, *Thinking with demons*, 163–4.
[106] Rueff, *The expert midwife*, 55–61 (irregular pagination).
[107] Platter, *A golden practice of physick*, 171–2.

More emphatically, in the seventeenth century, Theophile Bonet concluded his discussion of the qualities of aphrodisiacs by stating that 'Aphrodisiacks take away also that impotency that is caused by Witchery.'[108] He recommended that herbs traditionally used to ward off incantations, such as St John's wort, should be mixed with satyrion.[109] He also suggested that the shavings of a Goat's horn or a decoction of Columbine, to wash the genitals, would be good.[110] Furthermore, Bonet did not simply recite these remedies from a previous author's work, or from popular understanding; he claimed to know of their efficacy through experience. He told his readers that 'I my self have restored some bewitched and tied up in this manner by Aphrodisiacks alone, particularly by the stimulating ... Chocolad.'[111] Although Bonet advocated aphrodisiacs by signature, it is clear that he was not employing them in a ritualistic or superstitious way, but as physical medicinal substances. Indeed, the use of sympathy and the doctrine of signatures may also have appeased popular notions of cures for bewitchment, as John Webster had suggested would be beneficial. Several other medical writers advocated cures that were likely to have been understood through the doctrine of signatures and occupied the liminal space between natural function and wondrous marvel. *Medicina magica tamen physica: magical, but natural physick* (1656), by Samuel Boulton, encouraged the belief that its remedies contained occult virtues and worked through hidden means.[112] Yet despite claiming to relate magical cures, Boulton included a recipe designed to strengthen the seminal powers and make the consumer fruitful, which contained known heating aphrodisiacs such as cinnamon, cloves, musk and amber.[113] Thus even Boulton's magical remedies drew upon the natural properties of plants and animal substances to affect a cure. He further complicated the advice that he gave his readers by proposing that only those plants which bore the signature of a disease should be employed in its cure.[114] Similarly John Pechey (1673) stated that enchanted men who could not have intercourse with their wives, or who were able to but did not emit seed, should drink 'a draught of cold water that drops from the mouth of a young Stone-horse as he drinks' as it

---

[108] Bonet, *Mercurius compitalitius*, 695

[109] Ibid.

[110] Ibid.

[111] Ibid. Bonet also stated that he cured someone using *rotulæ* of *Minsicht*. However, I have been unable to establish what he is referring to, *rotulæ* can mean both a small wheel, and a genus of sea urchin.

[112] Samuel Boulton, *Medicina magica tamen physica: magical, but natural physic*, London 1656. Little is known about Boulton: ODNB, *s.v.* 'Samuel Boulton', accessed 5 Nov. 2009.

[113] Boulton, *Medicina magica*, 102–3. Boulton offered (pp. 103–4) a second cure for 'them that are barren of either sex' which was composed of Satyrion water, salt of Satyrion, ambergris and musk.

[114] Ibid. 117.

was 'very potent'.[115] A stone-horse was an un-castrated stallion. It is likely that this water was thought to pass the potency of the stallion to the drinker, enhancing his sexual prowess and generative capabilities. Although these remedies contained elements of mystery and the unknown, it is likely that medical authors categorised and understood them plainly within the order of the natural world.

Other authors of this period also suggested that aphrodisiacs were employed to cure this form of impotence. Scot, in his list of cures, stated that 'Sir Th. *Moore* hath such a cure in this matter, as I am ashamed to write, either in Latine or English: for in filthy bawdery it passeth all the tales that ever I heard. But that is rather a medicine to procure generation, than the cure of witch-craft, though it serve both turnes.'[116] The description given here, a medicine to procure generation, would suggest that Thomas More had utilised a particularly potent aphrodisiac to serve as a cure for this form of enchantment, which resulted in particularly bawdy behaviour, perhaps similar to the behaviour associated with the use of cantharides. However, it is possible that Scot was vilifying Thomas More, whom he viewed as an unreserved Catholic. By suggesting that More had a bawdy remedy for this form of impotence Scot was able to imply that he gave credence to these diabolical instances. Moreover, he was able to intensify the insult by suggesting that Thomas More transgressed the boundaries of acceptable sexual knowledge by knowing and using remedies that caused excessive sexual behaviours.

The consumption of aphrodisiacs to cure infertility witchcraft continued into the eighteenth century. The *Ladies physical directory* (1739) stated, with a degree of scepticism, that some women who did not immediately know the cause of their sterility called it 'occult'.[117] The author then explained that, 'an ingenious Physician, who makes the Animal Œconomy his Study, is expert in Anatomy, and who carefully searches into the abstruse Principles and Causes of Things may easily investigate their Causes, and readily conceive the best Method of removing them'.[118] It is clear that this author did not believe that witches had the power to interfere with the genitals. Therefore cases believed by the ignorant to be caused by *maleficia* had physical causes and could be treated as natural disorders. This would conceivably have resulted in the use of aphrodisiacs as a cure. In the same way, Peter Shaw in *The new practice of physick* (1753), having noted the popular recourse to amulets and counter-magic, also stated that 'External remedies have been used in all ages, for relief in this case.'[119] Once again this would imply that physicians did not treat infertility witchcraft as a separate disorder

---

115 Pechey, *The compleat midwife's practice enlarged*, 243.
116 Scot, *Scot's Discovery of witchcraft*, 64.
117 Anon., *The ladies physical directory*, 48.
118 Ibid.
119 Shaw, *The new practice of physick*, 459.

and continued to employ natural remedies to combat the symptoms with which they were faced, in this case through the application of external stimulants, such as balms and ointments.

Recorded cases

This form of witchcraft was rare in England. In 1540 Henry VIII's inability to consummate his marriage to Anne of Cleves was described as relative impotence, an inability to have sex with one particular woman, which was normally associated with witchcraft.[120] However, this was downplayed in public in favour of non-magical explanations. The two cases published in the seventeenth century suggest a similarly ambivalent attitude towards magic of this kind. Moreover they suggest that focusing on the body of the victim and a natural response were elements of actual cases, as opposed to theoretical discussions. The first prominent case was that of Frances Howard who in 1613 petitioned for an annulment from her husband Robert Devereux, third earl of Essex. They were married at a young age and consummation of the marriage had been postponed for three years while the earl travelled. However, on his return the relationship deteriorated and in seeking an annulment Frances suggested that although they had lain together her husband was unable to consummate their marriage.[121] She further alleged that the 'Earle hath had, and hath power and ability of body to deal with other women'; Frances thus drew upon the well-established idea that impotence magic only prevented men from approaching specific women.[122] The Lord Archbishop, most likely the archbishop of Canterbury, George Abbott, consequently suggested that 'the Earle of *Essex* might be imagined to be troubled with *maleficium versus hanc*'.[123] Another telling of the event, however, alleged that a man called Forman, on Frances's behalf, 'did use all the *Artifice* his *subtilty* could devise, really to imbecillitate the Earl; for no Linnen came near his body, that was not rinsed with their *Camphire compositions*, and other faint and wasting ingredients ... to debilitate his *seminal operations*'.[124] The author of this text called Forman a conjurer and juggler, suggesting that a diabolical influence encouraged the use of natural herbs to induce

---

[120] ODNB, s.v. 'Anne of Cleaves', accessed 22 July 2013.
[121] ODNB, s.v. 'Frances Howard', accessed 22 July 2013; Bacon, A *true and historical relation*, 2.
[122] Bacon, A *true and historical relation*, 2.
[123] Ibid. 6. The Latin translates approximately as 'magic against this' or 'magic towards this'. This may represent that the magic was intended to impede his relations 'towards' his wife.
[124] Arthur Wilson, *The history of Great Britain*, London 1653, 58. It is also cited in David Lindley, *The trials of Frances Howard: fact and fiction and the court of King James*, London–New York 1993, 102.

sterility.¹²⁵ Nonetheless the narrative focused on the natural cooling and lust dampening effects of a known anaphrodisiac. The implication of impotence alone, excluding any connotations of witchcraft, was potentially embarrassing for the earl, particularly given his social standing and position. This argument shifted the blame for sexual failure onto Frances herself, and so absolved Robert Devereux of any shortcomings. The arguments portrayed in the printed versions of this trial suggest a rather ambivalent attitude towards impotence bewitchment. Although those in the case accepted the possibility of witchcraft magic, others returned to natural explanations for his ailments that firmly situated the blame for his inability with his wife.

The second recorded case of infertility witchcraft also involved a family of high social standing. In about 1618 the earl of Rutland and his wife were bewitched by the Flower family – Joan, Margaret and Phillip Flower.¹²⁶ In the printed version of this case, *Witchcrafts, strange and wonderfull*, details are provided of how the witches carried out their spell but no mention is made of the specific physical effects that they produced.¹²⁷ According to the treatise the witches killed cattle, caused sickness in the earl's eldest son, and caused the earl and countess to suffer sickness and convulsions, which they quietly submitted to believing that they were corrections from God.¹²⁸ After this the witches' desire for revenge increased and they 'determined to keepe them from having any more children'.¹²⁹ Interestingly it is not clear whether the action that they took was designed to prevent sexual activity; what was important to the witches was that the fertility of the couple was impeded. At the time the earl of Rutland and his wife did not attribute this misfortune to witchcraft. However, during the trial, Phillip Flower provided details of the spell. She explained that her mother

> tooke wooll out of the said matresse, and a paire of gloves, which were given her by Master *Vavasor*, and put them into warme water, mingling them with some blood, and stirring it together, then shee tooke the wooll and gloves out of the water, and rubd them on the belly of *Rutterkin* her Cat, saying, the Lord and the Lady should have more children, but it would be long first.¹³⁰

The cat was believed to be the witches' familiar, which provided the power to induce sterility in the earl. Yet it is not clear whether the wool and gloves

---

¹²⁵ Wilson, *The history of Great Britain*, 57–8.
¹²⁶ The examinations in the publication of the trial are dated to 1618. However, the events are likely to have taken place before this date.
¹²⁷ Margaret Flower, *Witchcrafts, strange and wonderfull: discovering the damnable practices of seven witches, against the lives of certaine noble personages, and others of this kingdome, as shall appeare in this lamentable history*, London 1635.
¹²⁸ Ibid. sigs Bv–B2r.
¹²⁹ Ibid. sig. B2r.
¹³⁰ Ibid. sig. C2r.

were placed within the boundaries of the earl's house, perhaps suggesting that physically manifested enchantments were not a crucial factor in English cases. Nevertheless, the glove and mattress wool, items from within the home that would have been in contact with the victim's body, may have ensured that the spell acted specifically upon the intended couple. Furthermore, the mattress wool would have been symbolic of the marital bed in which the couple should have conceived their children. The wool may therefore have guaranteed that it was the couple's generative abilities that were impeded.

The spell in this instance was not intended to cause permanent sterility; an unusual element as impotence witchcraft was often identified by its permanence.[131] Here, the temporary nature of the spell is the only detail provided about the intended results: the effects on the body were not described. What is clear is that the Flower women aimed to impede conception, not the ability of the earl and his wife to engage in sexual intercourse. Unfortunately no mention is made in this record of whether the earl and his wife sought treatment for their infertility. Instead the author records that God protected the earl and stopped the witches and the devil from afflicting him and his wife any further.[132]

These two cases both involved families from the upper classes who would have possessed a strong desire to conceive an heir who would inherit the title and lands associated with the family. By preventing these couples from conceiving the witches harmed the future of their family's position. The Rutland case is notably different from that of Frances Howard as both partners were afflicted by a party external to the couple. Nevertheless, the shame and embarrassment that accompanied both trials was perhaps very similar. In the printed narratives of these cases no mention is made of the practical application of remedies, and so it is difficult to establish whether the trend seen in the medical literature was a part of 'actual' cases of infertility magic.

Early modern society believed that there were a variety of ways in which magic and witchcraft could interfere with the generative system and cause infertility. Spells and enchantments, notably the ligature, or tying of knots, and the placing of an enchanted object within the boundary of a house were most commonly believed to cause these impediments. While many readers of texts on this subject would not have understood the intricacies of how the spell was supposed to affect the body, numerous spells were designed to induce erectile dysfunction, impede sexual pleasure and desire and prevent the flow of seminal fluid. The concern shown in the literature, and the rare English examples of infertility bewitchment, was directed towards the inexplicability of the disorder. However, the inexplicable nature of some aspects of this practice drew medical writers, and others, towards the corporeal aspects of this issue and its similarities to natural infertility. Discussions of bewitch-

---

[131] Kramer and Sprenger, *Malleus maleficarum*, 60.
[132] Flower, *Witchcraft, strange and wonderfull*, B2r.

ment were clearly framed within a naturalistic and humoural understanding of the body until the eighteenth century when the sexualised elements of maleficia were disregarded. The indistinct boundary between natural actions and magical effects, and the reliance upon the humoural understanding of the body, thus created a context within which medical writers and demonological scholars could advocate the use of natural sexual stimulants for the treatment of impotence in all its forms, including that induced by magic. Medical writers thus suggested several Galenic and sympathetic cures that were believed to either protect the body from witchcraft or remove the effects of an infertility enchantment. Given the rising scepticism concerning the power of witches, particularly in relation to magic affecting the generative organs, and perhaps the stigma of shame and powerlessness attached to this form of maleficia, it is plausible to assume that many who believed themselves to be a victim of witchcraft would have employed natural aphrodisiacs as a cure. In this way they could hope to avoid any association with the illicit cause of their disease.

The natural response of medical authors raises further questions about and complicates ideas about the prevalence of counter-magic in post-Reformation England. Keith Thomas has suggested that many men and women turned to the ritualistic remedies offered by cunning folk in the wake of the Reformation. However, the attempts by medical writers to demarcate the relevance and efficacy of natural medicaments in cases of infertility bewitchment may have influenced popular practice. The ability of medical writers to offer these substances suggests some measure of acceptance. Hence it may have been that post-Reformation society did indeed absorb cautions about the illicit nature of counter-magic. Although the evidence provided by these sources only allows us to glimpse the means that were utilised to restore the sexual potency of those afflicted with magical sterility, what is clear is that in this particular area, at least, the focus was predominantly on using recognised natural remedies to restore sexual ability and fertility.

5

Aphrodisiacs, Miscarriage and Menstruation

'THE Signs of this Disease are manifest; for such as are Barren, either bear not at all, or very seldom, and they breed but Weak and Tender Children.'[1]

Although discussions of barrenness and infertility were centred on the moment of conception, this was not viewed in isolation. Overall it was the inability of women, and men, to produce children that medical writers and practitioners were attempting to correct. There were two particular elements of the female body and reproductive process that had to be managed in order for a couple to demonstrate their fertility through living offspring. The first of these was menstruation, which was acknowledged to be of vital importance to the process of generation. Without adequate menstruation women were thought to be incapable of conceiving or nourishing the foetus *in utero*. Indeed medical writers discussed at length whether women were fertile and could have children before menarche (the onset of menstruation): Nicholas Culpeper for example asserted that 'They are called by some Flowers, because they go before Conception, as flowers do before fruit.'[2] It was imperative, as this chapter will demonstrate, that adequate menstrual bleeding was established before a couple could proceed to the process of generation. The second area of concern for medical writers was the potential for miscarriage. Conceiving a child was only the first step in bearing children. Medical writers throughout the period addressed the precarious state of the pregnant body and lamented that '*many sad and incommodious things are wont to happen to women with child*'.[3] These two medical conditions were understood to be part of the reproductive process and bounded the moment of conception. This chapter will consider the ways in which aphrodisiacs were understood in discussions of menstruation and in miscarriage, and will demonstrate that early modern sexual stimulants had a much broader role to play in the maintenance and regulation of sexual health than simply encouraging sexual behaviour near to the moment of conception.

---

[1] Salmon, *Systema medicinale*, 237.
[2] Culpeper, *Culpeper's directory for* midwives (1676 edn), 67–8.
[3] A. M., *A rich closet of physical secrets collected by the elaborate pains of four several students in physic*, London 1652, 1.

Provoking menstruation and provoking desire

Menstrual blood and the process of menstruation were considered to be central to a woman's reproductive potential. Non-menstruation could be an indicator of both ill health (it was related to numerous female ailments) and of pregnancy. Across the early modern period printed medical texts and manuscript collections contained numerous emmenagogues, remedies to 'provoke the courses', 'provoke the flowers' or 'promote the menses'. These were designed to rectify ill health by stimulating a flow of humours from the body. However, they have, as will be shown below, often been discussed in relation to contraceptive practices; they had the potential to be used to remove a pregnancy before it had become established. Nonetheless, it is evident that within the humoural framework these drugs had similar virtues to aphrodisiacs. They were also often given alongside aphrodisiacs and other fertility remedies. It will be argued here that viewing these remedies in conjunction with sexual stimulants demonstrates that menstrual provokers were an important first step in ensuring the fertility of the female body.

Many historians, such as Angus McLaren, Edward Shorter and John M. Riddle have identified herbs, and other emmenagogues such as iron filings, as a clandestine form of abortifacient, designed to remove an untimely or simply unwanted pregnancy.[4] In 1989 Roy Porter argued that during the long eighteenth century many remedies which 'promised to remove "female obstructions", and to procure, or renew menstruation' were actually substances that could be used to induce abortion.[5] Similarly Tim Hitchcock explained that birth control in eighteenth-century England included a variety of practices.[6] Of these, he wrote that

> Abortion of one sort or another was certainly the form of birth control spoken of most frequently. Throughout the early-modern period recipes for medicines to 'bring down the flowers', or to regulate menstruation, were a common component of any herbal or recipe book, and could certainly be obtained from the local apothecary.[7]

---

[4] McLaren, *Reproductive rituals*, 102–6, and '"Barrenness against nature": recourse to abortion in pre-industrial England', *Journal of Sex Research* xvii/3 (1981), 224–37 at p. 231. McLaren did acknowledge that some women used these simply to cure amenorrhea. See also Edward Shorter, *A history of women's bodies*, Harmondsworth 1984, 181–8; John Riddle, 'Oral contraceptives and early-term abortifacients during classical antiquity and the Middle Ages', *P&P* cxxxii (1991), 3–32 at pp. 11–23; and Laura Gowing, 'Secret births and infanticide in seventeenth-century England', *P&P* clvi (1997), 87–115 at p. 97.
[5] Porter, *Health for sale*, 148.
[6] Hitchcock, *English sexualities*, 52; Lawrence Stone, *The family, sex and marriage in England, 1500–1800*, London 1990, 266–7.
[7] Hitchcock, *English sexualities*, 52.

Once again Hitchcock made the assumption that the purpose of such medications was contraceptive. More recently Laura Gowing in *Common bodies* (2003) and Sarah Toulalan in *Imagining sex* (2007) have both stated that 'women's knowledge of the female body and its reproductive capacities included awareness (and use) of herbs and potions to prevent pregnancy, as well as techniques for "unblocking" the courses, or menstrual periods.'[8] These works do not completely disregard the ability of emmenagogues to promote conception; but they more frequently portray them as a means of procuring abortion.

The focus upon the abortive potential of these remedies may in part reflect the tendency of feminist and women's history to investigate abortion in early modern England as a means of demonstrating women's agency over their own bodies. For example, in *Blood, bodies and families* Patricia Crawford stated that 'as a method for preventing birth, abortion was successful. It was not a crime before the quickening of the child, and was under female control'.[9] Additionally she noted that women's agency in this case was not necessarily subordinate to male medical authority with women able to use physicians to provoke an abortion under the guise of restoring menstruation.[10] Similarly Gowing mentioned that the knowledge associated with inducing abortions could be guarded by early modern women as a part of female sexual knowledge.[11] The difficulty in assessing the true extent of abortion practices in early modern England has allowed for this interpretation which reads between the lines. This, combined with the desire to discover histories specifically about women, their bodies and their actions has allowed this interpretation of emmenagogues to become popular. Finally, Angus McLaren concluded in *Reproductive rituals* that 'The numerous references to abortifacient herbs provides evidence that they were not only widely available, but frequently' used.[12] That is, the sheer number of references to emmenagogues in both early modern manuscripts and printed works has contributed to the way in which they have been interpreted.

Several scholars have also focused on the social anxieties about single women and young maids of the early modern period when considering these drugs. They have aligned their interpretations of emmenagogues with the copious stories of the seduction of young vulnerable women by their masters or fellow servants, and the frequent suggestions of immoral women destroying the fruit of their wombs, found in both literary and medical works. This places the consumption of emmenagogues within a context of desperation which would lead women both to practise abortion and conceal its presence under

---

[8] Toulalan, *Imagining sex*, 74; Gowing, *Common bodies*, 47, 120.
[9] Crawford, *Blood, bodies and families*, 71.
[10] Ibid. 34.
[11] Gowing, *Common bodies*, 47.
[12] McLaren, *Reproductive rituals*, 106.

the guise of menstruation.¹³ This approach, however, downplays the wide range of unmarried and married women that sought to regulate their reproductive bodies. Moreover, it marginalises the widespread concern, found in medical and popular literature, for fertility and childbearing. Although the seduction of young women almost certainly led some to seek an abortion, it is important to temper this view. Martin Ingram's work suggests that between 1570 and 1640 illegitimacy rates were relatively low across England.¹⁴ He has also shown that the occurrence of master and servant sexual relationships was decreasing across the period.¹⁵ At first glance Ingram's work might suggest that many single women were aborting their unwanted pregnancies, causing a low birth rate for illegitimate children. However, he also noted that this may not have been the whole story. He explained that although savin and other potions were perhaps employed, it is also possible that a sizable portion of pregnancies terminated naturally; low levels of nutrition and poor standards of hygiene would have reduced the chances of a pregnancy surviving.¹⁶

The absence of a more nuanced approach to interpreting these substances, especially in studies of early modern England, is particularly surprising as Etienne van de Walle has emphatically argued that women in many geographical and historical settings have sought to manipulate their menstrual flow to promote fecundity.¹⁷ In 'Flowers and fruits', which traces Greek and Roman medicine through to the early modern period, van de Walle examined the emmenagogues listed in herbals and demonstrated their role in tempering the womb and promoting conception, as well as attempting to outline the level of practical application associated with these drugs.¹⁸ Moreover, van de Walle and Elisha Renne believe that Riddle, McLaren and others overstated the evidence when they accepted that many emmenagogues were simply used as abortifacients.¹⁹ Van de Walle's suggestions have encouraged new interpretations of these remedies. In her detailed examination of the original Hippocratic corpus of gynaecological recipes, Laurence Totelin argued that ingredients identified as abortive or expelling drugs could also be used in

---

[13] Gowing, 'Secret births and infanticide', highlights the difficulties of single early modern women when they fell pregnant. See also McLaren 'Barrenness against nature' 225–8, and *Reproductive rituals*, 89–94.

[14] Ingram, *Church courts, sex and marriage*, 19.

[15] Ibid. 265.

[16] Ibid. 159.

[17] Etienne van de Walle and Elisha P. Renne (eds), *Regulating menstruation: beliefs, practices, interpretations*, Chicago 2001, p. ix.

[18] Etienne van de Walle, 'Flowers and fruits: two thousand years of menstrual regulation', *Journal of Interdisciplinary History* xxviii (1997), 183–203 at pp. 192–3, 195–201.

[19] Van de Walle and Renne, *Regulating menstruation*, p. xiv.

compositions that furthered sexual health.[20] She has concluded that in the Hippocratic recipes helping conception was a very similar process to purging and regulating the menstrual cycle.[21] In this situation she has argued that 'it is important not to interpret all Hippocratic gynaecological purges as abortions'.[22] Similarly Monica Green, for the medieval period, has argued that, 'we must be very cautious in assuming, as Riddle does, that every substance identified as an emmenagogue was used with the *intention* of preventing pregnancy or aborting one already begun. Infertility was and remains a problem for a considerable number of women'.[23] All of these scholars have highlighted that within a context where the promotion of fertility, rather than its suppression, was key a more nuanced approach should be taken to understanding these remedies.[24]

Early modern medical practice was founded fundamentally upon the teachings of Hippocratic and Galenic medicine, and continued to follow many beliefs expounded throughout the medieval period. Hence it is apparent that the medical framework of the early modern period would not automatically have categorised these substances as negative. Accordingly, Gowing has suggested that a more nuanced interpretation of abortive and emmangogic drugs is necessary for this period. Following the revelation that women used these substances for abortive purposes, she concluded that

> while these phrases [, such as bringing down the terms,] can be read as euphemisms for early abortion, in the context of early modern prescriptions of pregnancy, they make sense on their own terms: what we recognise as early pregnancy could be perceived, then, as an obstruction in the menstrual flow which might, or might not, eventually lead to a quick child.[25]

Cathy McClive has also conducted extensive research into the attitudes towards menstruation of medical practitioners in early modern France. She has demonstrated that physicians and medical writers were concerned about menstrual regularity: physicians attempted to rectify and restore vicarious menstrual bleeding (superfluous blood that could not escape through the uterus and so left the body through the anus, nose or ears) to ensure women's

---

[20] Laurence Totelin, *Hippocratic recipes: oral and written transmission of pharmacological knowledge in fifth- and fourth-century Greece*, Leiden–Boston 2009, 214, 219.
[21] Ibid. 216.
[22] Ibid. 217.
[23] Monica H. Green, 'Review of John M. Riddle, *Eve's herbs*', *Bulletin of the History of Medicine* lxxiii/2 (1999), 308–11 at p. 309.
[24] Idem, 'Bodies, gender, health, disease: recent work on medieval women's medicine', in *Studies in Medieval and Renaissance History: Sexuality and Culture in Medieval and Renaissance Europe* l (2005), 1–46.
[25] Gowing, *Common bodies*, 120.

fertile potential.²⁶ Finally, Bethan Hindson, in her discussion of Elizabethan attitudes towards menstruation, adopted a more flexible interpretation of medical attempts to promote menstrual bleeding. Even though she stated that bringing on the courses was used as a euphemism for abortion in seventeenth-century midwifery manuals, she went on to note that in many cases medical purges and expulsions were part of a complex understanding of the health benefits of menstruation – where absent menstruation was a symptom of some severe illnesses and disorders.²⁷ These health benefits included fertility.

Menstruation and fertility

The female generative organs were a mysterious entity in the early modern period. Menstruation and menstrual blood, in particular its qualities and its role in reproduction, were debated throughout the period. Most medical authors believed that menstrual blood provided the nutrition given to the baby during gestation. Conversely, there were those who thought that menstrual blood was the woman's contribution to the forming foetus: it was shaped and invigorated by the male semen at the point of conception to create the new life. Thus, whether it was a nutritious superfluity or the woman's contribution to conception, menstrual blood was regarded as a key component in the reproductive process.

Joan Cadden has suggested that for medical men in the Middle Ages menstrual retention was the most prominently discussed cause of female barrenness, with John of Gaddesden actually placing it 'first in his list of ten intrinsic causes'.²⁸ During the early modern period general medical texts and midwifery manuals often expressed the concern that a lack of menstruation could prevent a woman from conceiving a child. Similarly Cathy McClive has demonstrated in her studies of early modern France that despite the complex and ambiguous understanding of menstrual blood the link between menstruation and fertility was accepted.²⁹ In England the concern was widespread and persistent across the period. Jakob Rueff argued in 1554 that the state of a woman's menstrual flow affected the health of her entire body.

---

[26] Cathy McClive, 'Menstrual knowledge and medical practice in early modern France, c. 1555–1761', in Shail and Howie, *Menstruation*, 81–2, 86.

[27] Hindson, 'Attitudes towards menstruation', 95–6. See also Barbara Traister, '"Matrix and the pain thereof": a sixteenth-century gynaecological essay', *Medical History* xxxv/4 (1991), 436–51 at p. 440, and John Christopoulos, 'Abortion and the confessional in Counter-Reformation Italy', *Renaissance Quarterly* xlv/2 (2012), 443–84 at p. 446.

[28] Joan Cadden, *Meanings of sex difference in the Middle Ages: medicine, science, and culture*, Cambridge 1993, 250.

[29] McClive, 'Menstrual knowledge and medical practice', 86.

He wrote 'so that her body be of a sound and healthfull constitution, [it] ought naturally to be Purged and cleansed from this superfluous matter every moneth'.[30] Furthermore, he lamented the effect of absent menstruation upon the generative organs, stating that 'every woman deprived of these Flowers, I say, of this purging in her due season by the course of Nature, can neither conceive, nor ingender, being like unto an unfruitful and a barren man, destitute and deprived of the same vertue, and faculty of ingendring'.[31] It is clear from Rueff's statement that a lack of menstruation was not simply detrimental to fertility but entirely destructive to the ability to bear children. This sentiment was echoed by Alessandro Massaria in 1657. He wrote of the danger to the woman's body if her monthly purgation was suppressed, stating that 'there followes to that Woman much peril and many sicknesses'.[32] He also continued to caution his readers that 'if there be a perpetual suppression of the Terms, then it plainly shows such a Woman to be absolutely barren'.[33] Again, Massaria emphasised that the effects of not experiencing proper menstruation were severe: it could mean the total loss of a woman's reproductive capacity. He also explained that this disorder could be intimately linked with the humoural constitution, as Rueff also implied; the deficiency could be caused by obstructions, excessive fatness or leanness or coldness of the womb, which made the woman dull, drowsy, and slowed her pulse.[34] It is not surprising then, that many remedies which served to correct this suppression were similar in nature to aphrodisiacs that heated the body.

Across the period medical writers continued to extol the necessity of menstruation to fertility. The consistency of this belief once again demonstrates the continuity and longevity of the humoural model and traditional medical knowledge in this area. While authors could be divided about the purpose of menstrual blood, it was consistently acknowledged that a complete lack of this blood, or the retention of this blood within the body, causing an internal excess, was damaging to the delicate humoural balance of the reproductive system. In the late seventeenth century Jane Sharp addressed her readers' concerns about what hindered conception. Instead of outlining the damaging effects of not having a proper menstrual flow, she wrote 'let such as desire to have children, look to it that their courses come down orderly, and be well coloured, for then there is no fear but such women will be easie to conceive'.[35] By explaining the role of menstruation in this way Sharp may have encouraged her readers to provoke the courses themselves. This text explicitly states that the woman must make certain that her 'courses come

---

[30] Rueff, *The expert midwife*, 11.
[31] Ibid.
[32] Massaria, *De morbis fœmineis*, 16.
[33] Ibid. 20. Massaria reasserted his concerns later in his work, at p. 118.
[34] Ibid. 20.
[35] Sharp, *The midwives book*, 180.

down orderly', overtly encouraging active measures to reinstate the proper menstrual cycle. In the eighteenth century medical writers continued in the same vein, agreeing that menstruation was crucial for fertility.[36] Several treatises even went as far as to connect menstruation with the ability to feel sexual desire: the anonymously authored *Ladies physical directory* explained that without menstruation 'then the natural sparkling Briskness of the Blood and Juices is wanting, the lively desirous Faculty is spoiled, neither is the womb fit to receive the spirituous *Effluvia* of the Masculine *Semen*, that Conception might follow'.[37] The consensus amongst these authors across the period about the centrality of menstruation and menstrual blood to fertility makes it all the more surprising that the role of emmenagogues in improving fecundity has not been more thoroughly examined for the early modern period. The unified message of these descriptions provided readers of medical treatises with a context in which the provocation of absent menstruation would have been framed within the treatment of barrenness.

The connection between menstruation and sexual pleasure was expounded in several other eighteenth-century medical treatises. In drawing this connection these authors helped further to establish the context within which emmenagogues could be recommended alongside aphrodisiacs in order to further fertility and encourage intercourse. For example, John Marten explained in 1709 that

> A depravation of the *Menstrual Flux*, or difficulty of the *Terms*, is a Disease also that hinders Procreation, and sometimes abates the Pleasure of Copulation, because they are troubled upon that Indisposition with a pain in the Belly, shooting Pains in the Loins, Groins, Head-achs, Stomach-ach, &c which unfits them for Coition.[38]

Similarly, in 1729, in the vernacular version of the first tract dedicated to discussing menstruation, John Freind related that some had been of the opinion that menstrual blood affected the pleasurable nature of sex. He explained:

> The final Cause of the Menses, is agreed by Authors to be, either to render Woman more apt for Conception, or to afford Nutriment to the Fœtus. Those, who embrace the former Opinion, assert the menstruous Flux to be necessary upon the following Account, that the Blood being purged from any filth or dregs, may both the more forcibly excite the Women to Coition, and also more happily receive the Seed.[39]

---

[36] Bracken, *The midwife's companion*, 28; Foster, *The principles and practice of midwifery*, 28.
[37] Anon., *The ladies physical directory*, 48; Ball, *The female physician*, 70.
[38] Marten, *Gonosologium novum*, 107, 112.
[39] Freind, *Emmenologia*, 4.

It is clear in this excerpt that the blood assisted pleasure once it had been purged and cleansed. Although this understanding may only have related to those who saw menstrual blood as an excrement that had to be purged from the body, it does suggest that promoting the expulsion of menstrual blood from the body was viewed as directly related to increasing both sexual pleasure and the fertility of a woman's body.

Even without a direct link to sexual pleasure, it is apparent that medical authors across the period understood that proper and regular menstruation was a crucial element of the fertile female body. The explanations that these writers presented to their readers emphasised the role of the humoural constitution in the correction of this problem and the link to increased sexual desire and pleasure. Thus it is unsurprising that these authors advocated the use of aphrodisiac substances to invigorate the body with heat and pleasure alongside substances that would encourage a natural flow of blood. Within this context many women would have viewed remedies to provoke menstruation as falling entirely within the realms of sexual health practice, rather than simply as a way to remove an unwanted pregnancy.

In addition simply to noting the importance of regular monthly purgation, medical writers also recommended recipes that could be used to purge the body of this retained blood and revive a natural and timely cycle. While it is clear that these remedies could be easily utilised for the purposes of removing a blockage or an obstruction, in the form of a newly developing foetus, it is also apparent that they were designed to improve the fertility of the reproductive organs. As Laurence Totelin demonstrated, within the Hippocratic understanding of fertility purges were often viewed as the first step towards ensuring a conception.[40] Early modern authors almost unanimously offered a selection of purging remedies for those women wishing to stimulate menstruation. In the sixteenth century Jakob Rueff explained as a part of his 'generall Precepts serving for the curing of the barrenness' that

> let women observe and consider the complexion and state of the Matrix, and let them warily marke their Termes, lest in the time when they issue forth, or when they are cleared from them, they use an inconvenient diet, but that rather they use most especially such things which are knowne to have an expulsive vertue and force to expell out of the body: such as are parsley, Stone-parsley, Fennel, the herbe which the Germans call commonly Pimpinella, with the like herbes and roots of the same nature and quality.[41]

He thus explicitly recommended purgation of the female body and the use of expulsive herbs to promote fertility. Similarly, in the seventeenth century, Alessandro Massaria's first recommendation was for the remedy hiera picra,

---

[40] Totelin, *Hippocratic recipes*, 217.
[41] Rueff, *The expert midwife*, 49.

which was much recommended to purge excrements from the body.[42] He also listed several stronger purgative medicines which could be utilised should the initial treatments prove unsuccessful.[43] It is possible that stronger remedies were more likely to be viewed by both contemporary readers and historians as abortifacients but were not necessarily produced only for this operation; they could still be used for medicinal sexual health purposes.

These purging remedies which cleansed the womb of corrupt humours continued to be advocated into the eighteenth century. In *Gonosologium novum* (1709) John Marten acknowledged that strong purgative medicines could be required in the cure of barrenness caused by blocked menstruation. Moreover, his recommended purge used a particularly powerful and dangerous aphrodisiac, cantharides. This example thus implies that these two types of substance shared common virtues. In the treatise Marten wrote that to cure this disorder 'universal Remedies which evacuate upwards or downwards, must be first given', after which he listed several purging medicines.[44] He followed this with the caution that

> some Cases have been so inveterate, as that for the better forcing and opening of these obstructed Passages, we have been forc'd to have recourse to *Cantharides*, both inwardly and outwardly apply'd; for such a Distemper, unless in time remov'd utterly spoils Procreation, and much impedes Copulation.[45]

Here the remedy was designed solely with the promotion of generative health in mind. Even though cantharides could conceivably have been used to purge a foetus from the body, Marten did not invoke the familiar warnings offered to pregnant women across the period by medical writers discussing potentially abortifacient substances. His purges were explicitly understood and described solely within the framework of curing barrenness.

Purges designed to stimulate the monthly courses and restore the fertility of the womb were also discussed and recorded by female manuscript-writers. As with the published examples, it is clear that these could have been adopted for a more sinister use. Because they were recorded in domestic recipe books they could have been accessed in a clandestine manner, without the necessity of visiting a doctor or apothecary. This potentially allowed them to be used to remove a pregnancy before it was discovered by those around the woman. Often, though, these remedies were recorded with the names of women who could attest to their efficacy. One recipe in the manuscript attributed to Lady Ayscough (1692) is annotated with 'Probat Mrs Sadler' and 'Probat, Mrs Hone'.[46] It can be assumed that these women would not have been willing

---

[42] Massaria, *De morbis fœmineis*, 21.
[43] Ibid. 24–35.
[44] Marten, *Gonosologium novum*, 109.
[45] Ibid.
[46] WL, MS 1026, 140.

to allow their names to be ascribed to an abortifacient with the suggestion that they had used it; evidently they had used the remedy for health purposes. Moreover, to view emmenagogues exclusively within the context of contraception is to undermine the importance of fertility to early modern women. Several examples from the seventeenth and eighteenth centuries highlight the link between provoking the terms and encouraging conception. They each described the remedy in terms of helping barren women to conceive. One of the most descriptive was recorded in Lady Ayscough's manuscript. The documented recipe was supposed to 'cleanse the Reines' (kidneys), and so the urinary passages, thereby conforming to the stereotypical abortifacient virtues – the removal of obstructions or impurities in the womb.[47] It contained parsley seed as its primary ingredient, which was known to provoke the terms; consequently it can be assumed that this was one of its aims.[48] Nevertheless, the title given to this remedy indicated that purging was not viewed as a detrimental or damaging course of action: it was meant to be cleansing and as such would leave the body in a purer, more fertile state. The recipe was very complex, preventing it from being a suitable quick fix for an unwanted pregnancy. Moreover, in addition to the parsley it contained numerous provokers of lust, including hazelnuts and the 'pythe' of an oxe back; this suggests that it was indeed supposed to cleanse and then invigorate the womb, bringing it to a more pleasurable and fertile state.[49] The final notation about the remedy further emphasised its place as a part of reproductive health practices: this remedy was 'Prob[atum est]: by Mrs Hone who being 4 years without issue being married conceived with Child upon ye taking thereof.'[50] Another similar example was recorded in the recipe collection of the Boyle family. One family member recorded 'A Course of Physick much tryed and approved to purge the womb of superfluous humours and to promote Conception in Barren Women.'[51] This included many herbs noted for their ability to provoke the terms, including pennyroyal, madder, calamint and savin. Yet it is once again clear that provoking the terms was

[47] Ibid. 104.

[48] Ibid. Information on the virtues of parsley from Nicholas Culpeper, *The English physician: or an astrologo-physical discourse of the vulgar herbs of this nation: being a compleat method of physic*, London 1652, 188.

[49] WL, MS 1026, 104. 'Pythe' may have referred to the spongy interior of the bulls organs, particularly its horns, or the substance occupying the spinal cord. It was a common medical theory that semen was produced in the brain and travelled to the testicles through the spinal column. This would suggest that the doctrine of signatures was employed here to pass on the potency of the ox to the woman consuming the decoction: *OED*, *s.v.* 'pythe', accessed 9 Aug. 2013.

[50] WL, MS 1026, 104.

[51] WL, MS 1340, fo. 35v.

thought to be beneficial to the generative faculty of the womb.[52] Thus the evidence presented in both printed medical works and manuscript collections shows that provoking the terms was viewed as a form of cleansing purge which purified the womb and made it ready for conception.

The way in which these manuscript recipes were recorded meant that they were inherently open to interpretation. Not all recipes included specific directions for creating the remedy. As Elaine Hobby and Catherine Field have shown, the quantities of herbs used in recipes was left to the discretion of the woman, meaning that the recipe and her knowledge of the effects that these herbs would have in various quantities was developed through a working system of testing.[53] By utilising these remedies in their own practice, it was expected that most women would have an intimate knowledge of the plants required and the amounts in which they were effective. As a result historians have been able to interpret these compounds as being heavily dominated by the expulsive faculties of the emmenagogue ingredients. Nonetheless women at the time would have been able to interpret these recipes in the way that suited their circumstances: those needing an abortion could do so by including a more potent ratio of emmenagogues. Conversely, those seeking to cleanse and purge the womb to improve fertility could do so by balancing out the strength of potential abortifacients with the stimulating properties of provokers of venery.

Emmenagogues and aphrodisiacs

In addition to the presence of evidence that linked potential abortifacients and emmenagogues with the treatment of barrenness, many purgative substances shared humoural virtues with potent aphrodisiacs. According to the 1655 edition of the *Pharmacopoeia londinensis*, the humoural composition of many emmenagogues classified them as hot and dry, usually to the second or third degree. Culpeper described hot in the second degree as 'something hotter than the Natural temper of man', while those of the third degree were 'more powerful in their operations'.[54] This category included herbs such as capper roots, carline thistle, flower-de-luce, dittany, fennel, cassia lignea, angelica and mugwort, which were able to bring on the courses.[55] Being hot and dry were also very common qualities of the provokers of lust listed in

---

[52] Ibid. Another example is recorded in the book of Mary Doggett whose plaster for the back 'being laid to ye belly of a woman it causeth her Terms and makes her apt to conceive': BL, MS Add. 27466, fo. 39v.

[53] Hobby, *The virtue of necessity*, 167; Field, '"Many hands hands"', 56–7.

[54] Culpeper, *Pharmacopoeia londinensis* (1655 edn), 346.

[55] Ibid. 3, 3–4, 5, 7–8, 14, 18, 19. Other examples are maudlin, 17; water calamint, 21; ground pine, wild chamomile and germander, 23; sampier, 24; clary 28; common horehound, 30; thyme, 37.

the *Pharmacopoeia*. This probably reflects the similar nature of the causes of these two disorders, predominantly being attributed to excessive coldness and moisture in the body. It may also reflect the fact that these two disorders were seen as commonly linked: suppressed menstruation caused barrenness, thus they should be treated with similar herbs. The number of herbs listed with these virtues in the text also suggests that this was not an uncharacteristic or exceptional occurrence. The provokers of lust listed as hot and dry in the second, third or fourth degree included: elecampane, eryngo, galangal, southernwood, rocket, garden cresses and cloves.[56]

Furthermore, numerous herbs and other medicaments were described as able to provoke lust as well as menstruation. At the beginning of the period Anthony Askham's herbal informed its readers that both mugwort (motherwort) and frankincense cleansed the womb and helped conception.[57] Very few of Askham's medical practices are known: only his published works on astrology, herbal lore and almanacs.[58] As such, the extent to which he applied this knowledge is uncertain. However, Askham does again highlight that purgatives were not necessarily viewed as a means to destroy conceptions. In the seventeenth century many more examples of herbs with these counterpart virtues can be identified. John Gerard wrote in the *Generall historie of plantes* that saffron stirred up fleshly lust and brought down the flowers.[59] Similarly, John Pechey's late seventeenth-century herbal recorded that garden clary provoked the courses and stimulated venery.[60] Arabella Atkyns's *Family magazine*, a text supposed to influence domestic practice, also stated that cresses were 'very warm, provoke to venery ... and promote the menstrual flux'.[61] These examples highlight the fact that medical writers recognised the diversity of virtues of these herbs. Although the versatile nature of these plants might appear contradictory, humoural medicine allowed for substances to act in a variety of ways. Totelin has identified that the dual use of plants was not contradictory to readers of the original Hippocratic corpus.[62] Consequently these plants could be used for entirely separate purposes. They may have been employed solely to empty the womb without the associated ideas of enhancing procreation, but they were just as likely to be used to promote conception and cure barrenness.

---

[56] Ibid, 6, 7, 16, 26, 32, 41.

[57] Askham, *A lytel herbal*, sigs Fiiir, Fviv.

[58] *ODNB*, *s.v.* 'Anthony Askham', accessed 29 May 2013.

[59] Gerard, *Generall historie of plantes*, 151–4. See also Culpeper, *Pharmacopoeia londinsensis* (1655 edn), eryngoes, 6; valerian 2, 10; carrot seeds, 42; chickpeas, 43.

[60] Pechey, *The compleat herbal* (1694 edn), 48. See also John Pechey, *The compleat herbal of physical plants*, London 1707, 54–5, 165. John Riddle also identified many emmenagogues which could also be reconsidered as aphrodisiacs: *Contraception and abortion*, 85.

[61] Arabella Atkyns, *The family magazine: in two parts*, London 1741, 8.

[62] Totelin, 'Sex and vegetables', 536.

APHRODISIACS, MISCARRIAGE AND MENSTRUATION

Although many emmenagogues could also be identified as provokers of lust, certain herbs were notoriously described as abortifacients during this period, particularly pennyroyal, savin and ergot, although others, including hellebore, chervil and bistort were also commonly listed.[63] Nevertheless, even when these herbs were employed it may have been to induce fertility, rather than abortion or miscarriage. Compound remedies which were thought to promote the terms often contained numerous herbs of varying qualities and could include provokers of lust. In these cases the aphrodisiacs included were either thought to be simultaneously stimulating menstruation, or were necessary to ensure that the rectified state of the womb, which now experienced regular monthly purgation, was fertile and desiring of a conception.

The most striking remedies which combine several emmenagogues and several aphrodisiacs can be found in the *Pharmacopoeia londinensis*. This treatise included a description of 'Dr Stephens water', which in numerous manuscript recipe collections was described as a remedy for barrenness.[64] Here however, it was described as 'profitable for women in labor' and 'it provokes the terms'.[65] Even though this particular description did not state that the remedy was a cure for barrenness, this water, when viewed as a recipe, seems to contain a half and half split of aphrodisiacs and abortifacients:

Take of Cinnamon, Ginger, Galanga, Cloves, Nutmegs, Grains of Paradice, Seeds of Annis, Fennel, Caraway, of each one dram; Herbs of time, Mother of Time, Mints, Sage, Penyroyal, Pellitory of the wal, Rosemary, flowers of red Roses, Chamomel, Origanum, Lavender, of each one handful; infuse them twelve hours in twelve pints of Gascoign wine.[66]

Although, as has been established, some of the provokers of lust included in this remedy were also believed to stimulate menstruation, several more were included which were not thought to affect menstrual flow. Moreover, the aphrodisiac substances were clustered together, perhaps suggesting that this was the way in which they were expected to work. Thus, although this recipe would potentially have provoked the terms and induced uterine contractions during labour, under the humoural model in which many of these substances raised heat and desire it may also have been intended to stimulate the fertility and pleasure of the womb, inducing it to conceive a child.

Another electuary that was designed to open the womb and restore menstruation also contained more aphrodisiacs than emmenagogues. This remedy was described as able to provoke the terms, strengthen the stomach

---

[63] McLaren, *Reproductive rituals*, 104.
[64] Culpeper, *Pharmacopoeia londinensis* (1655 edn), 100; WL, MS 373, fos 55v–56r; MS 7818, 13; BL, MS Sloane 3842.
[65] Culpeper, *Pharmacopoeia londinensis* (1655 edn), 100.
[66] Ibid.

and aid the distribution of nourishment around the body, effects that would have aided the womb to bear children.[67] The remedy contained

> Cinnamon fifteen drams; cassia Lignea, Alicampane-roots, of each half an ounce: Galanga, seven drams; cloves, long Pepper, both sorts of cardamoms, Ginger, mace, Nutmegs, Wood of Aloes, of each three drams: Saffron one dram: Sugar five drams: Musk two scruples.[68]

The prominence of sexual stimulants in these recipes strengthens the suggestion that many of these potentially abortive substances were thought to have a beneficial effect on the generative system, reflecting the multiplicity of values that early modern medicines could have. Similarly, some substances which were promoted without a list of ingredients were also thought to work in this two-fold manner. The 'English PILLS FOR THE SCURVY' described in an anonymous text on *Some particular rebellious distempers* were advocated for their ability to 'Cure Barrenness effectually, whether the fault be in the Man or Woman; they exalting the Generative Faculty, cleansing and strengthning the Spermatick Vessels, resisting all Foulness and Infection in the Act of Generation; bring down the Terms in Women and Maids.'[69] Once more the emphasis here was upon the ability of the medicine to promote the generative faculty and enliven the reproductive organs: provoking menstruation was a part of this process, not a separate action. These emmenagogic remedies were not presented in medical literature as a covert way of designating abortions, but rather held a legitimate place in medical treatments for infertility.

The grave concern surrounding the issues of barrenness and menstrual regularity in early modern England, combined with the close links between emmenagogues and provokers of lust, suggests that many of the recipes prescribed to restore natural menstruation were indeed recommended for this purpose. Furthermore, the combination of abortifacients and aphrodisiac simples in compound recipes shows that these recipes were frequently understood within, and designated as a part of, sexual health treatments to rectify, and purify, the state of the womb, reinvigorating it as a fertile organ. It may also be that these aphrodisiacs were included to ensure that once the womb had been returned to a fruitful state the woman was also encouraged to enter into copulation and so conceive a child. It is apparent that these recipes were sometimes misappropriated and utilised as covert abortions to remove unwanted or inconvenient pregnancies, but this interpretation should not completely overshadow the descriptions, understandings and warnings

---

[67] Ibid. 237.

[68] Ibid; Massaria's treatise also listed a strong purging remedy that contained several stimulating substances including, sperage, fennel, cinnamon, parsley, fennel seed, yellow rape seed, caraway, galangal and saffron: *De morbis fœminis*, 28.

[69] Anon., *An account of the causes of some particular rebellious distempers*, London 1670, 1, 12.

of danger to women with child which were originally attributed to them. Instead many of these simples and compound remedies should be accepted on their own terms and understood as occupying a position of versatility within early modern sexual health medicine.

Aphrodisiacs and the prevention of miscarriage

For many medical writers, both before and during the early modern period, the problem of fertility was not solely that of conceiving a child. In examining the Middle Ages Joan Cadden has noted that while medieval scholars focused on the moment of conception, in general they thought about the process of generation broadly, encompassing sterility, conception, miscarriage, stillbirth and deformed children.[70] In the early modern period authors also followed this mode of describing barrenness.[71] Ensuring that a foetus survived after the initial conception was another facet of the same sexual health problem. In his study of sixteenth- and seventeenth-century pregnancy, Michael Eshleman has argued that the possibility of a miscarriage influenced every facet of pre-natal care.[72] Given the intertwining of conception, pregnancy and birth it would perhaps be expected that aphrodisiacs were employed throughout the period of gestation to support a healthy and fertile environment in the womb. Yet this was not so. Medical writers implied that the promotion of conception and the maintenance of pregnancy were connected, and several authors suggested that sexual stimulants could be used for this purpose. Nevertheless, they did not usually advocate them in these circumstances. Instead only a few select stimulants, rather than the full range of aphrodisiacs, were repeatedly noted in remedies designed to prevent miscarriage.

Medical writers during this period did not rigidly and consistently use the term miscarriage to discuss the loss of a foetus during pregnancy. Often the term abortion, or early term abortion, was also used to describe this event.[73] It is important to note that abortion at this time did not necessarily mean the deliberate termination of a pregnancy. Many authors used the terms abortion and miscarriage interchangeably: Jane Sharp's *Midwives book* for example stated that 'There are abundance of causes whereby women are

---

[70] Cadden, *Meanings of sex difference*, 250.
[71] Massaria, *De morbis foemineis*, 102; Culpeper, *Culpeper's directory for midwives* (1676 edn), 132; Shaw, *A new practice of physick*, 452.
[72] Michael K. Eshleman, 'Diet during pregnancy in the sixteenth and seventeenth centuries', *Journal of the History of Medicine and Allied Sciences* xxx (1975), 23–39 at p. 37. Angus McLaren also discussed protection from miscarriage: *Reproductive rituals*, 46–9.
[73] This was also true in the Italian context: Christopoulos, 'Abortion and the confessional', 445.

driven to abort, or miscarry'.[74] Similarly, in a 1690 edition of the popular sex manual *Aristotle's master-piece*, in a chapter on 'What a woman ought to observe after conception', the author noted that 'in the first two Months after Conception, Women are very subject to Miscarriage, because the Ligaments are weak, and soon broken ... But if notwithstanding Signs of Abortion or Miscarriage appear, let her lay Toast dipt in Tent ... to her Navel'.[75] Some texts did suggest that there was a difference between the two: a later edition of *Aristotle's master-piece* described how

> Many Physicians there are, and indeed most of them make difference between a Mischance and Abortion: The former of which, say they, is when there is a Conception, but through the slipperiness or weakness of the Womb, it drops out e're any shape is contracted, being only a Rude unframed Mass, properly called the Rudiments of a Child, that shhuld [sic] have been, and a shadow of what was begun; but Abortion oft times shews the parts of the Infant perfectly composed.[76]

The author implied here that the two terms were interchangeable in vernacular usage but that trained physicians knew the distinction between the two. However, this may not have been the case as medical texts written by physicians did not always make this distinction: the English edition of Christopher Wirtzung's general medical treatise explained that conceptions and foetuses could be lost at different stages of the pregnancy but termed all of these 'an *Abortus*, that is, a mischance'.[77]

Thus it would appear that the terms miscarriage and abortion could be used interchangeably to describe the loss of a foetus during pregnancy. What these authors do suggest was of importance was the time at which this occurred. Although this did not change the label applied to the phenomenon, medical men were at pains to point out that a woman could lose either an unformed or a fully formed child. The descriptions that these writers provided of the various stages of foetal formation that could be disrupted and disturbed by a range of activities, diseases and shocks served to emphasise the precarious and perilous nature of pregnancy from the moment of conception through to the moment of birth.

---

[74] Sharp, *The midwives book*, 221.

[75] Anon., *Aristotle's compleat master-piece ... Displaying the secrets of nature in the generation of man*, London 1690, 39. Tent was a deep red Spanish wine of low alcohol content: *OED*, s.v. 'Tent', accessed 10 Apr. 2012.

[76] Anon., *Aristotle's master-piece* (1694 edn), 53–4. See also Hugh Chamberlen, *The accomplisht midwife*, London 1673, 129.

[77] Wirtzung, *The general practice of physicke*, 508. See also Sennert, *Practical physick*, 172.

Preventing miscarriage with aphrodisiacs

The information presented in vernacular medical texts relating to the prevention of miscarriage, as with many other areas of medical discussion, was heterogeneous and often contradictory. In particular, medical authors across the period were uncertain of the role that aphrodisiacs played in ensuring that pregnancy was successful. For many authors, the treatment for miscarriage once the warning signs of abortion had been established, seldom included provokers of lust, with more importance being ascribed to medicaments specifically thought to be virtuous in this situation, such as mugwort and tansy. These two plants were believed to enhance the state of the womb and ensure its continued health: tansy consumed phlegmatic and cold humours and strengthened the reins (kidneys) and the back, while mugwort eased inflammations and obstructions of the womb.[78] Nonetheless, authors did imply that aphrodisiacs could serve a function in ensuring the continued healthy state of the womb. Jakob Rueff, in *The expert midwife*, noted that the first method of preventing miscarriage was to identify before conception those women who were 'accustome to Abort' and to ensure that they were 'comforted and strengthened with convenient meat and drinke'.[79] This suggests that women could be given nourishment designed to enhance the health and fertility of the womb to ensure that it was well suited to carry a child to term. Yet Rueff also noted that once conception had occurred women should avoid 'immoderate *Venus* [and] unsaciable lust', which were acknowledged causes of untimely miscarriage.[80] Rueff's advice was not necessarily contradictory, but rather a caution about timing; aphrodisiacs were allowable before conception but not afterwards, and especially not when the signs of abortion had been identified. Furthermore, he may have been cautioning against excess. The consumption of aphrodisiacs could strengthen and nourish the body, but eating too many could have encouraged the woman to engage in intercourse, which was considered potentially harmful to the developing foetus.[81]

That aphrodisiacs might have been employed to prevent miscarriage was also implied by John Sadler in *The sick woman's private looking glasse* (1636). Although little is known about Sadler and his medical practice, he claimed that his treatise presented women with an authoritative understanding derived from Galen and Hippocrates.[82] He argued that an imbalance of

---

[78] Culpeper, *The English physician*, 86, 225.
[79] Rueff, *The expert midwife*, 167.
[80] Ibid. 164–5.
[81] Sixteenth-century Italian theological texts also taught priests that sexual stimulation during pregnancy could result in the loss of an unfinished foetus: Christopoulos, 'Abortion and the confessional', 448.
[82] Sadler, *The sick woman's private looking glasse*, sig. A4v.

humours was often the cause of early abortion: 'Sometimes by humidity weakening the faculty that the fruit cannot be retain'd untill the due time: by drinesse or emptinesse, defrauding the childe of his nourishment.'[83] He further noted that women should avoid being fearful because it caused the heart to forsake the womb, thus allowing cold to strike it, and caused the ligaments retaining the baby to collapse.[84] The descriptions provided by Sadler bear a remarkable resemblance to the causes of barrenness examined in chapter 2. In this context Sadler's readers may have applied their knowledge of warming and strengthening aphrodisiacs to counteract these effects. Indeed, in *Reproductive rituals*, Angus McLaren concluded that miscarriage remedies containing cinnamon, nutmeg, sugar and eggs were often intended to warm and strengthen the patient.[85] Similarly, Ulinka Rublack has demonstrated that German midwives perceived anger and shock as hazardous to the foetus and subsequently offered remedies of saffron or cinnamon taken in wine.[86] Thus, the similarities between the causes of barrenness and the causes of miscarriage may have encouraged men and women to use the same aphrodisiac medications to augment and strengthen the womb in both scenarios.[87]

The role of aphrodisiacs in maintaining pregnancy remained unclear throughout the seventeenth century. In her 1671 midwifery treatise Jane Sharp exemplified the similitude with which these two areas of reproductive health could be viewed. Sharp offered a multitude of advice concerning the cure of barrenness in women. She suggested that 'before she be conceived with child, let her use means both by diet and physick to strengthen her womb, and to further conception'.[88] This course of physic included drinking 'wine that is first well boyled with mother of Tyme, for it is a precious thing', and consuming juniper berries every morning if the womb was too windy.[89] For those whose wombs were too moist she recommended galangal and cinnamon taken in muscatel and in more general terms she discussed the use of 'Oyl of Nightshade' and 'the Seeds of Mandrakes'.[90] While each of these remedies was theoretically well suited to enhancing fertility, this was

---

[83] Ibid 152.

[84] Ibid 152–3.

[85] McLaren, *Reproductive rituals*, 47.

[86] Ulinka Rublack, 'Pregnancy, childbirth and the female body in early modern Germany', *P&P* cl/1 (1996), 84–110 at p. 96. What is not clear from these discussions is whether aphrodisiacs were employed for their ability to create pleasure, which may have counteracted the negative influences of fear, anger and shock.

[87] Seventeenth-century handbill advertisements also frequently paired the treatment of miscarriage and barrenness: BL, 551.a.32.[21], [179], [206]; BL, C.112.f.9. [45]; C.112.f.9. [66].

[88] Sharp, *The midwives book*, 176.

[89] Ibid.

[90] Ibid. 176–7.

not the context in which this information was originally provided. Much of Sharp's work was derived from Nicholas Culpeper's *Directory for midwives* (1651).[91] In this instance she repeated, almost verbatim, Culpeper's chapter '*of Preventing Miscarriage*'.[92] Although this might seem to have been a misappropriation of the information, this is not necessarily the case. In his work Culpeper divided his recommendations for the treatment of women liable to miscarry into sections outlining the medications that could be given before pregnancy and during pregnancy, as Sadler had done. This suggests that Culpeper viewed the promotion of conception and the maintenance of pregnancy as very closely related. Sharp appears to have developed this attitude further by listing both of these sections as a means for ensuring conception and remedying barrenness. For Culpeper, preventing miscarriage inevitably meant strengthening the womb and ensuring conception, while for Sharp, guaranteeing conception undeniably included the prevention of miscarriage. Hence, the same instructions could be used for both barrenness and early miscarriage.

Aristotle's master-piece also offered a confusing amalgamation of ideas that potentially allowed for the use of aphrodisiacs in preventing miscarriage. Furthermore, this tract, like many other treatises, did recommend remedies that included provokers of lust. The longevity of this text (130 printings and up to forty-three editions had appeared by 1800 and further editions were reproduced into the twentieth century) and the fact that it was aimed at a wide audience, including those who purchased ballads and almanacs, also suggests that the ideas that it presented were to some extent popular.[93] The author's advice detailing how a woman should govern herself during her pregnancy implicitly promoted the use of sexual stimulants as a means of maintaining pre-natal health and preventing a miscarriage. The reader was informed that during gestation meats should be eaten in moderation and that 'the most wholsom Meats in this case are Pidgeons, Turtles, Larks, Partridges, Pheasants, Veal, Mutton, or any such Meat that is of good Juice, and contributing to kindly Nourishment'.[94] The majority of these foods were also described as aphrodisiacs, which provided nourishment that encouraged seed production and conveyed the lecherous qualities of small birds to the consumer. Indeed, *Aristoteles master-piece* listed aphrodisiacs in a similar

---

[91] Fissell, *Vernacular bodies*, 199; *The midwives book; or, The whole art of midwifry discovered by Jane Sharp*, ed. and intro. Elaine Hobby, Oxford–New York 1999, pp. xviii, xix.

[92] Culpeper, *A directory for midwives* (1651 edn), 147–78 (original in italics).

[93] Again I note my thanks to Mary Fissell for sharing information on the number of editions published. See also Roy Porter, 'The literature of sexual advice before 1800', in Porter and Teich, *Sexual knowledge*, 134–57 at p. 136, and Roy Porter and Lesley Hall, *The facts of life: the creation of sexual knowledge in Britain, 1650–1950*, New Haven–London 1995, 33–6.

[94] Anon., *Aristotle's master-piece* (1694 edn), 123–4.

language: 'such as are subject to Barrenness should eat such Meats only as tend to render them fruitful; and among such things are ... all Meats of good juice, that nourish well ... of which Faculty are all hot moist Meats' including pigeons, partridges, pheasants and sparrows.[95] Following this kind of recommendation, those seeking to prevent the onset of an early abortion could plausibly have reverted to foods known to enhance the state of the womb, including aphrodisiac substances.

Despite the suggestion that heating herbs and nourishing foods could prevent miscarriage, medicines in the early modern period were rarely specifics. Although they could have particular virtues that they were known for, they were also often multi-functional. In particular, remedies for the womb could be relevant in several related disorders, such as infertility and miscarriage. Aphrodisiacs were widely understood in the early modern period, appearing in medical texts, diaries and ephemeral literature, and may have been recognisable for these qualities; it was perhaps the clear association that these substances had with sexual stimulation and fertility that both suggested a use in miscarriage and ultimately prevented their application. Their use before conception was considered unproblematic as they improved the fertility of the womb and enhanced its potential to carry a child to term. Aphrodisiacs could also be used in moderation after conception to protect a pregnancy, but medical writers were much more cautious about suggesting this. Although a few authors thought that engaging in intercourse after conception was innocuous, most believed that sexual stimulation and activity could be dangerous to a pregnancy.[96] Thus, Jakob Rueff cautioned his readers that pregnant women should avoid 'immoderate *Venus* [and] unsaciable lust' because it could cause a miscarriage.[97] As with other excessive emotions such as anger, fear and joy that disrupted the blood flow to the womb and caused an abortion, sexual stimulation was a hazard in itself. More important, arousal could lead to sexual activity which, like dancing, horse riding and other vigorous exercises, was believed to loosen the bands which fastened the child to the womb.[98] Thus medical writers did not actually want to provoke lust after conception had occurred for fear that they would inadvertently cause a woman to miscarry.

In the eighteenth century the implicit acceptance of aphrodisiacs as either innocuous or beneficial to the prevention of miscarriage faded from medical texts. The *Ladies dispensatory* (1740) offered several remedies for miscarriage but these contained only a few provocative substances.[99] Similarly Jean

---

[95] Anon. *Aristoteles master-piece* (1684 edn), 11–12.

[96] Jane Sharp allowed that women could have sex while pregnant and conceive a second child as a result: *The midwives book*, 71.

[97] Rueff, *The expert midwife*, 164–5.

[98] Riverius, *The practice of physick*, 513.

[99] Anon., *The ladies dispensatory*, 242–7.

Astruc's *The art of midwifery* (1767) recommended a decoction of mugwort, oil of sweet almonds and a potion of plantain, milfoil, mastic, bistort and tormentil to prevent a miscarriage.[100] This rejection of nourishing and warming foods may have been influenced by the emerging sense of food and medicine as distinct entities.[101] Earlier in the period culinary and medicinal recipes often appeared side by side, in both manuscript and printed works, because all ingestible substances had a humoural virtue that would have an effect upon the body.[102] With the introduction of new chemical, Paracelsian, ideas about treatment in the seventeenth century printed works began to show evidence of a separation between food and medicines.[103] Reproductive medicine was to some extent resilient to change and innovation. Consequently, it might have been that the separation of food and medicines in this area was not apparent in the printed literature until the eighteenth century.

The absence of aphrodisiacs from eighteenth-century discussions of miscarriage was however tempered by the continued printing of older works that presented seventeenth-century, and even older, information to new audiences. Nicholas Culpeper's advice, which dealt with these two issues consecutively, was republished throughout the eighteenth century.[104] The consistent reliance of medical and midwifery treatises on traditional explanations of distempers and treatments also meant that ideas about the pregnant body that were prevalent in the seventeenth century continued to be espoused in the eighteenth century. *The art of midwifry* (1752) by George Counsell explained that in addition to the dangers of falls, bruises and frights, miscarriage could be induced by a humoural deficiency, 'from her natural Constitution being either too weak, moist, and slippery; or too dry and rigid.'[105] This suggests that, in addition to the perpetuation of older texts, newer midwifery treatises continued to understand miscarriage using the humoural framework. Readers encountering these traditional descriptions of miscarriage could have continued to utilise hot and nourishing herbs and foods in order to strengthen the body and prevent miscarriage. Counsell also suggested that 'you must help the Woman with proper nourishing and strengthening Drinks and Cordials' if the injury or distemper becomes unavoidable and the woman needs to expel her burden.[106] Here

---

[100] Astruc, *The art of midwifery*, 144–6. See also Ball, *The female physician*, 79–84.
[101] Field, '"Many hands hands"', 53.
[102] Ibid. 52.
[103] Lynette Hunter, 'Women and domestic medicine: lady experimenters, 1570–1620', in Lynette Hunter and Sarah Hutton (eds), *Women, science and medicine, 1500–1700*, Stroud 1997, 89–107 at p. 96.
[104] Culpeper, *A directory for midwives* (1701 edn), 97; *A directory for midwives*, London 1716, 97; *A directory for midwives*, London 1755, 89; *A directory for midwives*, London 1762, 97.
[105] George Counsell, *The art of midwifry: or, The midwife's sure guide*, London 1752, 162.
[106] Ibid. 163.

then nourishing and strengthening aphrodisiacs were also attributed a role in ensuring the safety and survival of the mother when an abortion did occur. As an extension of this practice some people may have employed heating, nourishing and strengthening foods to guarantee the survival of the mother through the difficult time of pregnancy.

Overall, when discussing the prevention of miscarriage, medical writers did not explicitly exclude the use of aphrodisiacs. Indeed they noted that conception and gestation were part of the same process of generation and that the body could be strengthened with aphrodisiacs before conception. Heating and nourishing the body in this way made it more likely that a woman would both conceive and carry the foetus to term. It was thus the inherent understanding that aphrodisiacs improved fertility that suggested that they could have a role in the prevention of miscarriage. Medical writers explained, in a similar manner to barrenness, that cold and weakness could cause miscarriage, which encouraged readers to rely upon those herbs and meats that were known to strengthen the womb and provide warmth and nourishment. Medical texts, therefore, created a context within which aphrodisiacs could be considered beneficial to the prevention of miscarriage, as a part of the wider understanding of generative health. Yet, recommendations for their use largely remained implicit.

Within this context, some authors explicitly described remedies for miscarriage that would have been considered to be sexually stimulating. In particular, several remedies contained nutmeg, cinnamon, or cloves, or a combination of these simples. Despite his intricate cautions regarding moderation, Jakob Rueff acknowledged that to dispel wind from the womb and thereby prevent miscarriage, a woman's meat should be continually seasoned with cinnamon, nutmeg, cardamom, ginger, pepper and saffron.[107] These were heating herbs and correspond with McLaren's findings that these remedies were designed to warm the patient. To make an unguent to be laid to the womb, John Sadler (1636) suggested that nutmeg, mace, cloves and the oil of spike should be combined with several other ingredients.[108] Even though Sadler's other recipes did not incorporate many aphrodisiacs, the use of these heating substances by Rueff and Sadler suggests a propensity for the use of nutmegs, cinnamon and cloves. This was repeated across the period; Lazarus Riverius' *Practice of physick* advocated applying to the navel heating herbs, such as anise seeds, fennel seeds, powder of nutmeg and powder of coriander, to remove dangerous wind from the womb.[109] Although these

---

[107] Rueff, *The expert midwife*, 172.

[108] Sadler, *The sick woman's private looking glasse*, 159. For other recipes containing few aphrodisiacs see pp. 157, 158.

[109] Riverius, *The practice of physick*, 516. See also John Pechey, *A plain and short treatise of an apoplexy, convulsions, colick, twisting of the guts, mother fits, bleeding at the nose ... and several other violent and dangerous diseases*, London 1698, 22.

examples imply that heating herbs had an accepted and sustained role, it is notable that these remedies focus upon discussing wind from the womb, and thus served a specific function. In this context the role of stimulants in dispelling wind was perceived to be of value even though they may also have induced potentially dangerous sexual desire.

The understanding of reproductive health presented in printed works was mirrored in the manuscript recipe books of the era. This was also the case for miscarriage. In these collections, remedies for barrenness and miscarriage were sometimes recorded in close proximity, and in proximity to other generative disorders such as greensickness and childbed pains. Jane Jackson's 'very short and compendious method of physic' recorded seven recipes for ensuring conception followed by one 'To Keepe her conceaving', which enhanced the retention of the seed.[110] Similarly, the collection attributed to Ann Glydd confined most of her discussion of women's disorders to a cluster of folios.[111] For others the treatments themselves were one and the same: Anne Brockman's collection documented a remedy 'To prevent Miscarring, & healp Conception'.[112] Even though this particular remedy included no known aphrodisiacs it shows that women at this time believed it was possible to prevent miscarriage using the same treatments that served to enhance fertility.

Several manuscript authors included certain aphrodisiacs in their remedies against miscarriage. These would, presumably, ensure that the womb was correctly heated to support a conception, and then the developing foetus, and strengthen the blood, which served as nutrition for the growing child. In the latter part of the seventeenth century, one recipe in the collection ascribed to Elizabeth Jacob remarked that those who were likely to miscarry, or had a pain in the back, should combine four ounces of white lead, eight ounces of white seris, two great nutmegs, half an ounce of cloves and mace in a pint of 'sallet' oil.[113] Similarly Johanna Saint John's 1680 recipe book recorded that to prevent miscarrying, half an ounce of cloves should be boiled in rose water to create a syrup, which should then be taken morning, afternoon and evening or 'when any fright or disorder happens to you'.[114] Lastly, an anonymous seventeenth-century recipe collection included a remedy for 'such as are subject to miscarry' that contained a pound of currants, an ounce of nutmegs and a handful of clary along with nip (probably nep mint) and pimpernel.[115] These recipes suggest, again, that it was common to include

---

[110] WL, MS 373, fo. 74r.
[111] BL, MS Add. 45196: hard travail at fo. 38r; greensickness at fo. 39r; hurt in travail at fo. 40r; greensickness at fo. 41r; prevention of miscarriage at fo. 43r.
[112] BL, MS Add. 45197, 59.
[113] WL, MS 3009, 68. Seris refers to either endive or succory: Dodoens, *A niewe herbal*, 569; Parkinson, *Theatrum botanicum*, 774, 776.
[114] WL, MS 4338, fo. 213v.
[115] WL, MS 635, fo. 12v.

certain recognised sexual stimulants, nutmeg and cloves, in recipes designed to prevent miscarriage.

The importance of heat to sustained generative health could also be acknowledged in other ways; heat was always connected to the idea of life through the understanding of the body's vital heat. 'The Midwife Pill' was recorded in the recipe book of Theodosia Henshaw, which she attributed to a 'Dr. Willoby'.[116] Although it is not clear what the exact effects of the remedy were thought to be, it was noted that having consumed the medicine the patient was to 'lye warme & quiet as long as shee can'.[117] Thus, it would seem that this remedy was intended to warm, relax and rest a pregnant woman. In addition to these instructions the remedy contained mugwort, a herb specifically used to prevent abortion.[118] Those creating remedies in the home perhaps sought to combine the effects of herbs that were known to stimulate the generative organs and those that were believed to prevent early miscarriage. This collector also included asafoetida and saffron in the compound, both of which were thought to be aphrodisiacs.[119] The inclusion of these ingredients implies that the remedy was designed to invigorate and strengthen the womb and that the virtues of aphrodisiacs were considered beneficial to pregnant women. However, despite demonstrating a tendency to include aphrodisiacs in their remedies, it is clear that these substances did not dominate the compounds. The recipes were supposed to keep the patient warm and so in a healthy, fruitful balance of humours. The aphrodisiacs included were not necessarily supposed to sexually stimulate the generative organs, once again suggesting that treatments to prevent miscarriage were concerned about the damaging effects of sexual stimulation during pregnancy.

Early modern medical theory did not very often advocate specifics in terms of medical treatments and the qualities of medical substances. In nearly every instance plants and other medicines were thought to have multiple virtues which, in all probability, changed according to the context of the disorder and the humoural state of the body. This is particularly apparent in early modern herbals, and may have influenced the ambiguous understanding of aphrodisiacs and their relationship to miscarriage. In some cases herbs were listed as being of great benefit to those experiencing barrenness, or a complete lack of childbearing: they were recommended to both enhance the chances of conceiving and of the child being carried to term. Although these examples are rare they demonstrate an understanding that aphrodisiacs could

---

[116] WL, MS 7849, fo. 43r.
[117] Ibid.
[118] Ibid.
[119] Ibid. Dodoens, *A niewe herball*, 217; Parkinson, *Theatrum botanicum*, 261, 1569; Pechey, *The compleat herbal*, 210.

be used as a treatment to strengthen the womb throughout pregnancy. They also demonstrate that medical writers acknowledged the versatile nature of these plants and remedies. John Gerard, surgeon and curator of the Royal College of Physician's physic garden from 1586, discussed the virtues of sage in 1633, noting that it helped to prevent miscarriage and that it would help a woman to conceive. Gerard wrote

> *Agrippa* and likewise *Aetius* haue called it the Holy-herbe, because women with childe if they be like to come before their time, and are troubled with abortments, do eate thereof to their great good; for it closeth the matrix, and maketh them fruitfull, it retaineth the birth, and giue[t]h it life, and if the woman about the fourth day o[f] her going abroad after her childing, shal drink nine ounces of the juyce of Sage with a little salt, and then use the companie of her husband, she shall without doubt conceiue and bring forth store o[f] children, which are the blessing of God.[120]

Here Gerard did not separate the two virtues of this herb. This echoed the ideas of some medical texts which advocated that women who were prone to miscarry undergo treatment before the conceiving a child. Nicholas Culpeper used a similar description for tansy in his *English physician* (1652). He stated that

> Dame *Venus* was minded to pleasure Women with Child by this Herb, for there grows not an Herb fitter for their uses than this is, it is just as though it were cut out for the purpose, the Herb bruised and applied to the Navil staies miscarriage, I know no Herb like it for that use; boyled in ordinary Beer, and the Decoction drunk, doth the like, and if her Womb be not as she would have, this Decoction will make it as she would have it, or at least as she should have it; let those Women that desire Children love this Herb, 'tis their best Companion, their Husband excepted.[121]

Again, this excerpt addressed conception and parturition as one aspect of fertility. However, tansy was not commonly recorded as an aphrodisiac. Other herbs were described similarly. The anonymously authored *An English herbal* advised that Ladies Mantle 'helps Conception, and prevents Miscarriage'.[122] Similarly John Parkinson's *Theatrum botanicum* advised readers that artichoke thistles 'cause them to goe their full time in good plight, and also is very good for those that doe not teeme or are barren, and cause fertilitie'.[123] Consequently, although it was rarely in reference to the properties of aphrodisiacs,

---

[120] Gerard, *General history of plants*, 766. See also Culpeper, *Pharmacopoeia londinensis* (1655 edn), 35; Parkinson, *Theatrum botanicum*, 54; Anon., *An English herbal: or, A discovery of the physical vertues of all herbs in this kingdom*, London 1690, 54.

[121] Culpeper, *The English physician*, 225.

[122] Anon., *An English herbal*, 41; John Archer, *A compendious herbal*, London 1673, 85.

[123] Parkinson, *Theatrum botanicum*, 974.

herbals suggested to readers that certain herbs, known to help improve fertility, were applicable for the prevention of miscarriage. Combined with the understanding that conception and miscarriage were aspects of the same sexual health issue, it therefore seems plausible that people wishing to prevent miscarriage would have used provokers of lust to keep the generative organs warm and fortified.

Although still comparatively rare, examples of this kind can also be found in eighteenth-century herbals. In the 1707 edition of *The compleat herbal of physical plants* John Pechey, a licentiate of the Royal College of Physicians from 1687, described eryngo in the following terms: 'The Roots of it candied are accounted excellent Sweet-meats, and are Provocatives to Venery ... And used in the form of a Cataplasm, and applied to the Belly, it prevents Abortion.'[124] In this case the plant was discussed in terms explicitly relating to its stimulating qualities and its ability to maintain the health of a pregnant woman: eryngo was a frequently discussed aphrodisiac throughout the period. Unlike the discussions of sage which only infrequently mention its aphrodisiac virtues, this example directly implies a correlation between enhancing sexual desire and the prevention of abortion. Others herbs strongly associated with sexual stimulation were also discussed. Joseph Miller (1722) stated that from salap, thought to be the dried root of a form of orchis, 'a Decoction is made, and drunk hot like Tea, being accounted analeptic and strengthening, to prevent Miscarriage, and like Satyrion Root, is supposed to be a Provocative to Venery'.[125] While it is clear that Miller viewed this root as an aphrodisiac, it was not mentioned by other authors in this manner. He did however relate it to the satyrion root, which was ubiquitously understood to be an aphrodisiac, and stated that he thought this was a form of orchis, which was very frequently remarked upon for its stimulating properties. Unlike the earlier examples these authors explicitly connected the sexually stimulating properties of these plants with their ability to prevent miscarriage. This again implies that early modern men and women would have connected these two aspects of sexual health, and believed that aphrodisiacs were a useful remedy for ensuring that a foetus was carried to term.

Even though medical writers appear to have been concerned about the dangers of sexual stimulation and the use of aphrodisiacs to treat miscarriage, these medicaments did appear in this context in non-medical literature. The anonymous late seventeenth-century humorous work *The ten pleasures of marriage* discussed the enjoyments and responsibilities that a husband could look forward to once a previously barren wife had managed to conceive.[126] In response to the wife's expected groaning and grunting, especially during the

---

[124] Pechey, *The compleat herbal*, 84; ODNB, s.v. 'John Pechey', accessed 9 Aug. 2013.
[125] Joseph Miller, *Botanicum officinale; or, A compendious herbal: giving an account of all such plants as are now used in the practice of physick*, London 1722, 385.
[126] Marsh, *The ten pleasures of marriage*, 85–102.

night, the husband was encouraged to provide himself with 'pure Aniseed, Clove, Cinamon-waters and good sack, that you may therewith be ready to strengthen and assist her'; in particular these were described as helping to combat dizziness and faintness.[127] The author therefore implicitly supported the idea that great pains should be taken to prevent any accident that could upset the pregnancy. It is plausible to read these foods as a means of ensuring that the pregnancy continued. The spices discussed in this work are reminiscent of the particular spices, such as cinnamon, cloves, aniseed and mace, advocated ahead of other aphrodisiacs by medical writers to prevent miscarriage. Later in the same chapter, the author outlined that if a fault did occur the midwife would be called, who would recommend 'ofttimes to eat a piece of bread and butter with either Caroway or Aniseed Comfits, use also Cinnamon; the first expels wind, and the second strengthens the heart; and they are both good for the woman and the child'.[128] While this text sought humorously to outline all of the difficulties and annoyances of married life, it does to some extent illuminate what people would have identified with as everyday practice.[129] The overt discussion of stimulants seen in this text implies that the use of aphrodisiacs throughout pregnancy to prevent an untimely abortion was an accepted part of popular medical practice, although it tells us very little about the actual use of these substances in this way.

The evidence presented in early modern medical texts, herbals, manuscripts and popular literature suggests that aphrodisiacs had the potential to be thought of as a comprehensive form of fertility care, enhancing the chances of conception and ensuring that the foetus survived to term. Many authors viewed conception and pregnancy as intimately connected parts of the generative process. It was believed that women who were likely to miscarry should undergo treatment before they conceived a child. This treatment operated on very similar terms to the treatment of barrenness by using substances that strengthened and warmed the womb thus ensuring that it was healthy and fruitful. This perhaps was not unusual given the flexibility of most early modern remedies – remedies that affected the womb were potentially considered useful in all disorders of the womb. Nevertheless, medical writers presented a muddled account of the role of aphrodisiacs in this treatment. It was believed that God had created particular medicines for each different pathology, including miscarriage, and so aphrodisiacs were not also

---

[127] Ibid. 87.
[128] Ibid. 97–8.
[129] John Harvey suggests that this work displays a particularly English sense of humour, exaggerated in reaction to Puritanism. Harvey contends that the piece is typical of its genre if read in the context of the post-civil war proliferation in didactic works and guide books of domesticity. See A. Marsh, *The ten pleasures of marriage and the confession of the new-married couple* (Navarre Society, 1922), introduction by John Harvey at pp. v–xiv.

required. Nonetheless, midwifery treatises, herbals and manuscripts to some extent promoted the idea of conception and miscarriage as related topics and advocated sexual stimulants as a means to prevent miscarriage. Several heating stimulants in particular were noted with regularity: cinnamon, cloves, and anise seed. Yet, at no point were these herbs discussed explicitly for their ability to arouse the generative organs. One reason why medical writers of the period did not explicitly promote the use of aphrodisiacs for the treatment of potential miscarriages was because of their concern over the ill-effects of sexual stimulation. Lust and intercourse posed a threat to the health of the foetus and could cause a miscarriage. The inherent ability of these substances to stimulate sexual desire and pleasure prevented them from being an entirely suitable remedy for miscarriage.

Aphrodisiacs had a distinct medical role in the treatment of reproductive disorders and in the regimen required to ensure reproductive health. Stimulants were employed in multifaceted ways to improve the fertility of the female reproductive system. Before conception a woman's body had to experience regular and adequate menstruation. Numerous recipes were offered to provoke this, which have traditionally been interpreted as a means of provoking an abortion. Yet these remedies often contained aphrodisiacs and as such can be read on their own terms as part of women's efforts to ensure their own fertility. After conception, aphrodisiacs had the potential to be utilised for the promotion of a healthy pregnancy and the prevention of miscarriage during the early modern period. The pregnant body had to be kept in balance, kept well-nourished and strong, kept warm, and kept free of wind, and this could be achieved through the use of remedies that contained aphrodisiac substances. However, this was never fully articulated or advocated by medical writers. One reason for this was that sexual stimulation itself posed a threat to the pregnant body and could only be experienced in moderation. Likewise sexual activity, if too vigorous, could disrupt the pregnancy and cause its termination. The use of aphrodisiacs in these recipes highlights that women, and men, were proactive in regulating their reproductive bodies. The agency of men and women over these issues has usually been constructed in relation to the suppression of fertility and limiting of family size. Yet it is apparent that men and women understood how they could improve their fertility and take active steps to ensure that they bore children.

The presence of aphrodisiac substances in these discussions also reminds us that it is important to consider the whole process of reproduction: the moments of conception, miscarriage, pregnancy and parturition were all significant in and of themselves, but they were inherently connected to the experiences that had gone before and came afterwards. A child may not have been born had not the parents taken steps to provoke menstrual bleeding, improve their fertility and encourage sexual activity, and consumed remedies to prevent miscarriage. Medical writers and their audience acknowledged that fertility was a complex issue that could require long term care and advised their readers accordingly. The acceptance of this amongst the wider populace and the willingness of readers and patients to act upon this advice further cement the centrality of fertility to early modern lives and to early modern sexuality.

Conclusion

Early modern medical treatises paint a picture of many men and women struggling to conceive and give birth to live children. This was more than just a medical issue: reproductive failure undermined the happiness and stability of marriages, cast aspersions on a woman's character and hindered a man in fulfilling his patriarchal role. Childlessness was seen as a sign of God's displeasure and in some cases was interpreted as resulting from diabolical interference. It was greatly distressing and medical writers lamented the pain and desperation that these couples experienced. They noted that women in particular followed in the footsteps of the biblical Rachel who cried out '*Give me Children or else I die*'.[1] Medical writers and practitioners attempted to ameliorate this condition by advocating a range of therapeutic strategies that would improve fertility. Fundamental to these treatments, based upon the conviction that sexual desire and pleasure were inextricably connected to generation, was the use of a diverse range of aphrodisiacs.

Ideas about aphrodisiacs were not static in this period. As anatomical discoveries changed the way in which the reproductive organs were understood certain aphrodisiacs were rejected as ineffective – both for stimulating lust and improving fertility. There were also shifts in the understanding of infertility. In particular there was a move across the period towards the use of gender/sex specific labels for infertility in women and in men. This initially would appear to support the theory, proposed by Thomas Laqueur, that early modern anatomists and medical practitioners gradually came to accept the fundamental differences between the male and female bodies by the late eighteenth century. Taken together with the descriptions of aphrodisiacs and their functions a much more complex and rich picture emerges. Notions of aphrodisiacs and their functions remained, throughout the period, rooted in the belief that sexual desire and fertility were similar in both sexes. Although specific physiological processes were acknowledged for each sex, like menstruation, it was overall believed that men and women could be given the same aphrodisiacs in order to increase their sexual drive and make them more fertile.

As well as supporting critiques of Laqueur's theory, the discrepancy between the labels used to discuss infertility and the basis upon which treatments were advocated suggests that greater attention needs to be paid to the relationship between medical theory and medical practice when considering the development of medical knowledge. Medical practice existed within a

---

[1] Sharp, *The midwives book*, 177.

competitive marketplace populated by a range of practitioners who drew on a variety of medical frameworks; humoural, chemical, sympathetic and empirical. It is perhaps unsurprising then that medical writers advocated medicines that would be recognisable and would appeal to a broad audience, even when the theory behind them had been questioned. Medical writers and practitioners were also likely to recommend remedies based upon empiricism alone. It is important therefore to consider more closely the role of medical practice in shaping the continued popularity of different medical theories. It is also important to consider the role of theory and language in the medical marketplace, in promoting both traditional remedies and innovative medicines.

The use of aphrodisiacs to treat infertility and impotence magic raises similar questions about medical practice in this era. It has been argued that many men and women turned to ritualistic treatments and cunning-folk when faced with a malady caused by maleficium. Yet, medical writers, in addition to promoting the use of prayer, repeatedly and definitely suggested that victims should not turn to ritualistic treatments associated with pre-Reformation practices but should use natural substances and aphrodisiacs to deal with infertility magic. This may suggest that there was a measure of divergence in the responses of the wider populace and the medical elite to instances of magically induced infertility. However, as this book has shown, knowledge about aphrodisiacs and their uses and, importantly, access to sexual stimulants was possible for a range of men and women. Consequently, the response to infertility and impotence magic found in the medical literature questions the extent to which people internalised post-Reformation warnings about the illicit nature of counter-magic. Faced with exhortations from the Church to avoid superstitious remedies and claims by medical writers that these problems could be solved naturally, it is plausible to assume that readers of medical texts may not have resorted to counter-magic as readily as scholars have sometimes assumed. More work may therefore need to be done to assess the extent to which people in this period responded to the advice of medical men and the Church.

Throughout this book I have shown that medical writers and the wider populace accepted that the male body could be infertile and could be treated for reproductive failure. This contradicts many previous investigations of early modern infertility, which stated, as Olwen Hufton did, that 'in all European societies the blame for a failure to produce offspring was, almost without exception, laid at the feet of the woman'.[2] The acceptance and widespread discussion of remedies that would serve to improve both male sexual and reproductive abilities contributes to a new interpretation of infertility, advocated by Helen Berry and Elizabeth Foyster, as affecting and being

---

[2] Hufton, *The prospect before her*, i. 177; McLaren, *Impotence*, 75.

experienced by both women and men.³ Although the physiologies of the male and female form meant that there were some sex-specific causes and cures of infertility, it is just as apparent that infertility was not inevitably or universally blamed on women. It is thus important for scholars to reassess their ideas about the place of infertility in the history of men's bodies, manliness and masculinity: both sexual and reproductive failure could affect men and could have a severe impact on their lives.

The focus of scholars on the history of contraception and abortive practices has partially obscured a much richer and more nuanced history of fertility regulation. There has been a tendency to view the history of contraception and the history of infertility as separate, affecting separate people in very separate ways. However, the appearance of aphrodisiacs in the recipes for preventing miscarriage and for promoting menstruation should encourage us to question this division and think about sexual health practices in a more integrated way. In this book it has been shown that men and women took active measures in order to have and to keep having children. Yet it is entirely plausible that over the course of one lifetime a woman or man may have wanted to both limit and promote their fertility. That domestic recipe books, ballads and newspaper advertisements all include aphrodisiac remedies shows that fertility regulation was not necessarily a hidden or secretive practice. These remedies were for both wives and husbands. By looking beyond the context of illicit pregnancy and the desperation associated with it we can see that married couples may have wanted children and then in later years sought to limit their fertility. Moreover, if they suffered the devastating effects of the high infant mortality level in early modern England, they may subsequently have changed strategy, again attempting to improve their fertility. Knowledge of the sexual and reproductive body and the medical substances that affected it was adapted and manipulated in order to suit individual circumstances.

Although this book has focused on the use of aphrodisiacs to enhance fertility, it should also be emphasised that the widespread presence of sexual stimulants in the medical and popular literature of the early modern period also has implications for how we consider the history of sexuality. Laqueur has argued that in the eighteenth century the female orgasm, and the importance of sexual pleasure, diminished in medical discussions of reproduction.⁴ Yet the use of aphrodisiacs to enhance fertility was recommended throughout much of the eighteenth century. This suggests that while the importance of the orgasm for conception may have been gradually declining this did not necessitate a complete rejection of sexual pleasure from the process of conception. The use of such treatments was based upon the premise that pleasurable sex was more procreative and that procreative sex was pleasur-

---

3 Berry and Foyster, 'Childless men', 158–83.
4 Thomas, 'Orgasm', 1–41.

able, a principle that continued to be influential throughout the eighteenth century.

The strong emphasis on pleasure in the medical understandings of generation also contributes further complexity to the idea that it was in the eighteenth century that a more liberal attitude towards sexuality was adopted.[5] Although the overall attitude towards 'illicit' sexual activity was changing, focusing only on these types of sex ignores the importance that sexual pleasure had always had in early modern understandings of legitimate sexual activity, and the freedoms that this may have provided for men and women. Traditionally sexual activity within marriage has been viewed as constrained by the understanding that sex had to be generative and was often entered into with the aim of conceiving a child. Or it was considered to be necessary, a 'due benevolence' that maintained domestic harmony and prevented sexual transgressions. These religious and moral injunctions were certainly condoned broadly in society. However, it would be a mistake to think that much sexual activity in the early modern period was not enjoyed or that people did not necessarily expect it to be pleasurable. The evidence from ballads and erotic literature demonstrates that the pleasurable nature of sex was fundamental to people's expectations of sexual activity. This was supported by medical theory which dictated that all sex and particularly procreative sex should be both the result of sexual desire and result in sexual pleasure. Moreover, it is evident that men and women understood that they could enhance the desire and pleasure that they experienced by consuming aphrodisiacs. These, of course, could be used for improper purposes: John Marten cautioned readers of *Gonosologium novum* in the early eighteenth century that 'Old Letchers thinking to improve their former Prowess, and Young Gallants willing to merit their Misses good Will, do oftentimes misapply those Medicines.'[6] Yet in general these substances were rarely considered to be inherently sinful or illicit. They were described without concern for their potential use in seductions or extra-marital sexual activity in medical treatises, herbals and ballads. Understanding aphrodisiacs thus provides clear evidence for the everyday definable and legitimate place of sexual pleasure within the Church's teachings on sex and in the minds of the wider populace.

As in modern society, these titillating foods were known to encourage people to have sex. They were thus a remedy for one of the main causes of infertility, a loss of libido or frigidity, often caused by a cold constitution of the body. However, unlike modern society, aphrodisiacs in early modern England were known to be more than just sexual curiosities or consumables. They reinvigorated, heated, inflated, salinated and stimulated seed production, all of which made the body more fertile. Aphrodisiacs thus became a

---

[5] Dabhoiwala, The *origins of sex*.
[6] Marten, *Gonosologium novum*, 50.

central and ubiquitous element of early modern sexual health practices. This understanding of sexual stimulants was not arcane knowledge circulated only amongst elite medical men with classical learning; it was a common part of popular medical theory appearing in domestic recipe books, ballads and erotic literature. It is apparent, therefore, that understandings of sexual stimulants are contextual, not, as previous investigations have suggested, dehistoricised. Lust and sexual pleasure are not analogous in all time periods but are understood within the social, religious and (importantly) medical discourses of any particular era; in the early modern period they were central to comprehending the functioning of the reproductive organs and the act of generation.

Bibliography

Unpublished primary sources

London, British Library
MS Add. 27466   Receipt book of Mary Doggett, 1682
MS Add. 45196   Receipt book of Anne Glydd, 1656
MS Add. 45197   Brockman papers, vol. 130, 1638, Anne Brockman
MS Add. 56248   Receipt book of Lady Mary Dacres, 1600s
MS Add. 57944   Cookery and medical receipts compiled and owned by Mary Glover, 1688
MS Egerton 2197   Receipts of Elizabeth Digby
MS Sloane 556   Medical receipts written by Anthony Lewes, from a book owned by Lady Marquee Dorset, 1606
MS Sloane 1367   Lady Ranelagh's choise receipts
MS Sloane 2485   Margaret Baker, collection of receipts, 1650–72
MS Sloane 3842   Elizabeth Butler's book, 1679
551.a.32 Collection of handbill advertisements
C.112.f.9. [45], [66]

London, Wellcome Library
MS 213   Mrs A. Carlyon, 'A booke of divers medecins, broothes, salves, waters, syroppes, and oyntments … anno domini 1606'
MS 373   Jane Jackson, 'A very short and compendious method of phisicke and chirurgery'
MS 635   Receipt book, seventeenth century
MS 751   Elizabeth Sleigh and Felicia Whitfield, 1647–1722
MS 1026   Lady Ayscough, 1692
MS 1340   Boyle family, c. 1675–c. 1710
MS 3009   Elizabeth Jacob and others, c.1654–85
MS 3712   Elizabeth Okeover and others, c. 1675–c. 1725
MS 4338   Johanna Saint John, 1680
MS 7391   English recipe book, seventeenth century
MS 7745   English recipe book, later seventeenth to early eighteenth century
MS 7818   Collection of medical receipts in English
MS 7849   Theodosia Henshaw, late seventeenth century
MS 7851   Elizabeth Browne, Penelope Humphreys, Sarah Studman and Mary Dawes, late seventeenth to early nineteenth century

Printed primary sources

Newspapers
The British Journal
The Daily Courant
Daily Gazetteer
Daily Post
General Advertiser
London Journal
Middlesex Journal or Chronicle of Liberty, London, England
Mist's Weekly Journal
Spectator
Weekly Journal or Saturday's Post
Whitehall Evening Post

Contemporary books and articles
A. M., *A rich closet of physical secrets collected by the elaborate paines of four severall students in physick*, London 1652

Anon., *The accomplish'd female instructor: or, A very useful companion for ladies, gentlewomen, and others*, London 1704

Anon., *An account of the causes of some particular rebellious distempers*, London 1670

Anon., *The apprehension and confession of three notorious witches*, London 1589

Anon., *Aristotle's compleat master-piece ... Displaying the secrets of nature in the generation of man*, London 1690

Anon., *Aristotle's manual of choice secrets, shewing the whole mystery of generation*, London 1699

Anon., *Aristoteles master-piece, or, The secrets of generation displayed*, London 1684

Anon., *Aristotle's master-piece: or, The secrets of generation displayed*, London 1694

Anon., *A cheap, sure, and ready guide to health: or, A cure for a disease call'd the doctor*, London 1742

Anon., *The compleat doctoress: or, A choice treatise of all diseases insident to women*, London 1656

Anon., *The compleat wizzard ... together with several wonderful instances of the effects of witchcraft*, London 1770

Anon., *The contented cuckold: or, The fortunate fumbler*, London 1686

Anon., *The crafty whore: or, The mistery and iniquity of bawdy houses laid open*, London 1658

Anon., *A discourse on witchcraft occasioned by a bill now depending in parliament*, London 1736

Anon., *An English herbal: or A discovery of the physical vertues of all herbs in this kingdom*, London 1690.

Anon., *The English midwife enlarged*, London 1682

Anon., *Fumblers-hall, kept and holden in feeble-court, at the sign of the labour-in-vain, in doe-little-lane*, London 1675

Anon., *Labour in vain: or, The taylor no man*, n.p. 1675–96

Anon., *The ladies dispensatory: or, Every woman her own physician*, London 1740

BIBLIOGRAPHY

Anon., *The ladies physical directory: or, A treatise of all the weaknesses, indispositions, and diseases peculiar to the female sex*, London 1739

Anon., *The ladies remonstrance; or, A declaration of the waiting-gentlewomen, chamber maids, and servant maids*, London 1659

Anon., *The lamenting lady*, London 1620?

Anon., *The life and conversation of Temperance Floyd, Mary Lloyd; and Susanna Edwards three eminent witches*, London 1687

Anon., *The London cuckold*, London 1685–8

Anon., *The magick of Kirani king of Persia; and of Harpocration; containing the magical and medicinal vertues of stones, herbs, fishes, beasts and birds*, London 1685

Anon., *The Norfolk stiff-rump: or The apple-dumpling eater*, London 1692

Anon., *A pleasant treatise of witches their imps, and meetings*, London 1673

Anon., *The practical part of love: extracted out of the extravagant and lascivious life of a fair but subtle female*, London 1660

Anon., *A remedy for the green sickness*, London 1678–80

Anon., *The scolding wives vindication: or, An answer to the cuckold's complaint*, n.p. 1689

Anon., *The sorrowful bride: or, The London lasses lamentation for her husband's insufficiency*, London c.1682–94

Anon., *The well-approved doctor: or, An infallible cure for cuckolds*, n.p. c. 1685–8

Anon., *The womans brawl* (title page and date missing), ed. Roger Thompson, in *Samuel Pepys' penny merriments: being a collection of chapbooks, full histories, jests, magic, amorous tales of courtship, marriage and infidelity, accounts of rogues and fools, together with comments on the times*, London 1976

Anon., *The women's complaint against tobacco: or, An excellent help to multiplication*, London 1675

Archer, John, *A compendious herbal*, London 1673

Arnaud de Ronsil, Georges, *Plain and easy instructions on the diseases of the bladder and urethra*, London 1763

Askham, Anthony, *A lytel herball of the properties of herbes newly amended and corrected*, London 1550

Astruc, Jean, *A treatise on all the diseases incident to women*, London 1743

Atkyns, Arabella, *The family magazine: in two parts*, London 1741

Bacon, Francis, *Sylva sylvarum: or, A naturall history in ten centuries written by the right honorable Francis Lo. Veralum Viscount St. Alban: published after the authors death, by William Rawley doctor of divinitie, late his lordships chaplaine*, London 1627

——— *A true and historical relation of the poysoning of Sir Thomas Overbury ... also, all the passages concerning the divorce between Robert, late earle of Essex, and the Lady Frances Howard*, London 1651

Ball, John, *The female physician: or, Every woman her own doctress*, London 1770

Barret, Robert, *A companion for midwives, child-bearing women, and nurses*, London 1699

Barrough, Philip, *The methode of phisicke, conteyning the causes, signes, and cures of inward diseases in mans bodie from the head to the foote*, London 1583

Bartholin, Thomas, *Bartholinus anatomy made from the precepts of his father, and from the observations of all modern anatomists, together with his own*, London 1663

—— *Bartholinus anatomy made from the precepts of his father, and from the observations of all modern anatomists, together with his own*, London 1668
Blankaart, Stephen, *A physical dictionary in which all the terms relating either to anatomy, chirurgery ... are very accurately explain'd*, London 1684
Blondel, James Augustus, *The power of the mother's imagination over the foetus examin'd*, London 1729
Bonet, Theophile, *Mercurius compitalitius: or, A guide to the practical physician*, London [1682] 1684
Boulton, Richard, *A compleat history of magick, sorcery, and witchcraft*, London 1715–16
Boulton, Samuel, *Medicina magica tamen physica: magical, but natural physick*, London 1656
Bracken, Henry, *The midwife's companion: or, A treatise of midwifery: wherein the whole art is explained*, London 1737
Buchan, William, *Domestic medicine; or, A treatise on the prevention and cure of diseases by regimen and simple medicines*, London 1772
Bunworth, Richard, *Homotropia naturae: a physical discourse, exhibiting the cure of diseases by signature*, London 1656
Carroll, Robert and Stephen Prickett (eds), *The Bible: authorized King James version with Apocrypha*, Oxford 1998
Chamberlen, Hugh, *The diseases of women with child ... written in French by Francis Mauriceau*, London 1672
Chamberlen, Peter, *Dr Chamberlain's midwifes practice*, London 1665
Chorier, Nicholas, *The dialogues of Luisa Sigea*, Paris [1660] 1890
Cock, Samuel, *A voyage to Lethe*, London 1741
Cook, John, *An anatomical and mechanical essay on the whole animal oeconomy*, London 1730
Cooper, Thomas, *The mystery of witch-craft*, London 1617
Copland, William, *A boke of the properties of herbes*, London 1552
Cotta, John, *The triall of witch-craft*, London 1616
Counsell, George, *The art of midwifry: or, The midwife's sure guide*, London 1752
Cowper, William, *The anatomy of humane bodies with figures*, London 1698
Croll, Oswald, *A treatise of Oswaldus Crollius of signatures*, London 1669
Crooke, Helkiah, *Mikrokosmographia: a description of the body of man*, London 1615
—— *Somatographia anthropine: or, A description of the body of man*, London 1616
Culpeper, Nicholas, *A directory for midwives: or, A guide for women*, London 1651
—— *The English physician: or, An astrologo-physical discourse of the vulgar herbs of this nation: being a compleat method of physick*, London 1652
—— *Pharmacopoeia londinensis: or, The London dispensatory*, London 1653
—— *Pharmacopoeia londinensis: or, The London dispensatory*, London 1655
—— *Culpeper's directory for midwives: or, A guide for women*, London 1662
—— *Culpeper's directory for midwives: or, A guide for women*, London 1676
—— *A directory for midwives*, London 1693
—— *A directory for midwives: or, A guide for women*, London 1701
Daneau, Lambert, *A dialogue of witches, in foretime named lot-tellers and now commonly called sorcerers*, London 1575
Danet, Pierre, *A complete dictionary of the Greek and Roman antiquities*, London 1700

BIBLIOGRAPHY

Davenport, John, *Aphrodisiacs and love stimulants: with other chapters on the secrets of Venus*, ed. with intro. and notes Alan Hull Walton, London 1965

Della Porta, Giambattista, *Natural magick by John Baptista Porta, a Neopolitane: in twenty books*, London 1658

Dodoens, Rembert, *A niewe herbal*, London 1578

Drage, William, *Daimonomageia: a small treatise of sicknesses and diseases from witchcraft, and supernatural causes*, London 1665

—— *Physical experiments: being a plain description of the causes, signes, and cures of most diseases incident to the body of man*, London 1668

Drake, James, *Anthropologia nova: or, A new system of anatomy describing the animal oeconomy ... volume one of two*, London 1717

Elyot, Thomas, *Bibliotheca Eliotae*, London 1559

—— *The castell of health, corrected and in some places augmented by the first author thereof*, second edn, London 1595

Ettmüller, Michael, *Etmullerus abridg'd: or, A compleat system of the theory and practice of physic*, London 1699

—— *Etmullerus abridg'd: or, A compleat system of the theory and practice of physic*, London 1703

Ferrand, Jacques, *Erotomania: or, A treatise discoursing of the essence, causes, symptomes, prognosticks, and cure of love, or erotique melancholy*, Oxford 1640

Flower, Margaret, *Witchcrafts, strange and wonderfull: discovering the damnable practices of seven witches, against the lives of certaine noble personages, and others of this kingdome, as shall appeare in this lamentable history*, London 1635

Foster, Edward, *The principles and practice of midwifery*, London 1781

Freind, John, *Emmenologia: written in Latin by the late learned Dr. John Freind: translated into English by Thomas Dale M.D.*, London [1703] 1729

Fuller, Thomas, *Pharmacopoia extemporanea: or, A body of prescripts*, London 1710

Gerard, John, *The herball or generall historie of plantes: gathered by John Gerard of London master in chirurgerie very much enlarged and amended by Thomas Johnson citizen and apothecarye of London*, London 1633

Gibson, Thomas, *The anatomy of humane bodies epitomized*, London 1682

Hartman, George, *The true preserver and restorer of health*, London 1682

Harvey, Gideon, *The family physician, and the house apothecary*, London 1678

Hill, John, *The useful family herbal: or, An account of all those English plants, which are remarkable for their virtues*, London 1754

—— *The British herbal: an history of plants and trees, natives of Britain, cultivated for use, or raised for beauty*, n.p. 1756

James VI of Scotland, *Daemonologie, in forme of a dialogue, divided into three books*, Edinburgh 1597

Johnson, Robert, *Praxis medicinae reformata: or, The practice of physick reformed*, London 1700

Johnson, Samuel, *A dictionary of the English language*, London 1755–6

Jones, John, *The mysteries of opium reveal'd*, London 1701

Keill, James, *The anatomy of the humane body abridged*, London 1698

—— *The anatomy of the humane body abridg'd*, London 1718

Kramer, Heinrich, and James Sprenger, *The Malleus maleficarum*, ed. and trans. Montague Summers, New York 1971

Le Dran, Henri-François, *Observations in surgery: containing one hundred and fifteen different cases*, London 1739

Lemnius, Lævinus, *The secret miracles of nature: in four books*, London [1559] 1658
—— *A discourse touching generation*, London 1664
Luisini, Luigi, *Aphrodisiacus: containing a summary of the ancient writers on the venereal disease*, London 1736
Lupton, Thomas, *A thousand notable things, of sundry sortes*, London 1579
Macky, John, *Memoirs of the secret services of John Macky Esq: during the reigns of King William, Queen Ann, and King George I*, London 1733
McMath, James, *The expert mid-wife: a treatise of the diseases of women with child, and in childbed*, Edinburgh 1694
Marsh, A., *The ten pleasures of marriage relating all the delights and contentments that are mask'd under the bands of matrimony*, London 1682
—— *The ten pleasures of marriage and the confession of the new-married couple*, intro. John Harvey (Navarre Society, 1922)
Marten, John, *Gonosologium novum: or, A new system of all the secret infirmities and diseases, natural, accidental, and venereal in men and women*, London 1709
Massaria, Alessandro, *De morbis fœmineis; the womans counsellor: or, The feminine physitian*, London 1657
Miller, Joseph, *Botanicum officinale: or, A compendious herbal: giving an account of all such plants as are now used in the practice of physick*, London 1722
Moreiri, Louis, *The great historical, geographical and poetical dictionary*, London 1694
Newton, Thomas, *Approoved medicines and cordiall receiptes*, London 1580
Paracelsus, *Paracelsus of the supreme mysteries of nature ... translated by Robert Turner*, London 1655
Paré, Ambrose, *The workes of that famous chirugion Ambrose Parey*, London 1634
Parkinson, John, *Theatrum botanicum: the theater of plants*, London 1640
Pechey, John, *The compleat herbal of physical plants*, London 1694
—— *The store-house of physical practice: being a general treatise of the causes and signs of all diseases*, London 1695
—— *A plain introduction to the art of physick*, London 1697
—— *The compleat midwife's practice enlarged in the most weighty and high concernments of the birth of man*, London [1673]1698
—— *A plain and short treatise of an apoplexy, convulsions, colick, twisting of the guts, mother fits, bleeding at the nose ... and several other violent and dangerous diseases*, London 1698
—— *The compleat herbal of physical plants*, London 1707
Pierce, Robert, *Bath memoirs: or, Observations in three and forty years practice, at the bath, what cures have been there wrought*, Bristol 1697
Platter, Felix, *A golden practice of physick*, London 1662
—— *Platerus golden practice of physick*, London 1664
Purmannus, Mattheus Gothofredus, *Chirurgia curiosa: or, The newest and most curious observations and operations in the whole art of chirurgery*, London 1706
Quincy, John, *Dr Carr's medicinal epistles*, London 1714
—— *Lexicon physic-medicum: or, A new medicinal dictionary; explaining the difficult terms used in the several branches of the profession*, London 1726
—— *Pharmacopœia officinalis & extemporanea: or, A compleat English dispensatory, in four parts ... the fourth edition*, London 1726
R. B., *The kingdom of darkness: or, The history of daemons, spectres, witches, appari-*

tions, possessions, disturbances, and other wonderful and supernatural delusions, mischievious feats, and malicious impostures of the devil, London 1688

Radcliffe, John, *Dr. Radcliffe's practical dispensatory, containing a complete body of prescriptions*, London 1730

Raynalde, Thomas, *The byrth of mankynd, otherwyse named the womans boke*, London [1545] 1552

Riverius, Lazarus, *The practice of physick in seventeen several books*, London 1655

—— *The practice of physick in seventeen several books*, London 1678

Roberts, Alexander, *A treatise of witchcraft*, London 1616

Ross, Alexander, *Arcana microcosmi: or, The hid secrets of mans body disclosed*, London 1651

Rubenhold, Hallie (ed.), *The harlot's handbook, Harris's list*, Stroud 2007

Rueff, Jakob, *The expert midwife: or, An excellent and most necessary treatise of the generation and birth of man*, London 1637

Sadler, John, *The sick womans private looking glasse wherein methodically are handled all uterine affects, or diseases arising from ye wombe*, London 1636

Salmon, William, *Systema medicinale, a compleat system of physick theorical [sic] and practical*, London 1686

—— *Botanologia; the English herbal or history of plants*, London 1710

Scot, Reginald, *Scot's Discovery of witchcraft*, London [1584] 1651

Sennert, Daniel, *Practical physick: the fourth book*, London 1664

Sharp, Jane, *The midwives book: or, The whole art of midwifry discovered*, London 1671

—— *The midwives book; or, The whole art of midwifry discovered by Jane Sharp*, ed. and intro. Elaine Hobby, Oxford–New York 1999

Shaw, Peter, *A new practice of physick: wherein the various disease incident to the human body are described*, London 1753

Smith, Henrie, *A preparative to marriage*, London 1591

Smith, William, *Nature studied with a view to preserve and restore health: containing an explanation of the animal oeconomy*, London 1774

Turner, William, *A new herball*, London 1551

Van Deventer, Hendrik, *The art of midwifery improv'd: fully and plainly laying down whatever instructions are requisite to make a compleat midwife*, London 1716

van Diemerbroeck, Isbrand, *The anatomy of human bodies*, London 1689

Venette, Nicholas, *Conjugal love reveal'd: in the nightly pleasures of the marriage bed, and the advantages of that happy state: in an essay concerning humane generation*, London [1696] 1720

Vesling, Johann, *The anatomy of the body of man: wherein is exactly described every part thereof in the same manner as it is commonly shewed in publick anatomies … translated by Nicholas Culpeper*, London [1653] 1677

Webster, John, *The displaying of supposed witchcraft*, London 1677

Williams, William, *Occult physick: or, The three principles in nature anatomized by a philosophical operation, taken from experience, in three books*, London 1660

Wilson, Arthur, *The history of Great Britain*, London 1653

Wirtzung, Christopher, *The general practice of physicke*, London 1605

Woolley, Hannah, *The accomplisht lady's delight in preserving, physick, beautifying, and cookery*, London 1675

Secondary sources

Amory, Hugh, 'British books abroad: the American colonies', in Barnard and McKenzie, *Cambridge history of the book*, iv. 744–52

Ankarloo, Bengt, Stuart Clark and William Monter, *Witchcraft and magic in Europe: the period of the witch trials*, London 2002

Barclay, Katie, '"And four years space, being man and wife, they loveingly agreed": balladry and early modern understanding of marriage', in Elizabeth Ewan and Janay Nugent (eds), *Finding the family in medieval and early modern Scotland*, Aldershot 2008, 23–33

Barnard, John and Maureen Bell, 'The English provinces', in Barnard and McKenzie, *Cambridge history of the book*, iv. 665–86

Barnard, John and D. F. McKenzie (eds), *The Cambridge history of the book, IV: 1557–1695*, Cambridge 2002

Behrend-Martinez, Edward, *Unfit for marriage: impotent spouses on trial in the Basque region of Spain, 1650–1750*, Reno 2007

Benninghaus, Christina, 'Beyond constructivism?: Gender, medicine and the early history of sperm analysis, Germany, 1870–1900', *Gender & History* xxiv/3 (2012), 647–76

Berry, Helen, *Gender, society and print culture in late-Stuart England: the cultural world of the Athenian Mercury*, Aldershot 2003

—— and Elizabeth Foyster, 'Childless men in early modern England', in Berry and Foyster, *The family in early modern England*, 158–83

—— and Elizabeth Foyster (eds), *The family in early modern England*, Cambridge 2007

Black, Jeremy, *The English press in the eighteenth century*, London 1987

—— *Culture in eighteenth-century England: a subject for taste*, London–New York 2005

Blaen, Tom, 'The popular use of "precious" stones medicinally in early modern Scotland', in Georganta, Collignon and Millim, *The apothecary's chest*, 83–95

Bloch, Ivan, *Sexual life in England past and present*, London 1958

Bostridge, Ian, *Witchcraft and its transformations, c. 1650–c. 1750*, Oxford 1997

Cadden, Joan, *Meanings of sex difference in the Middle Ages: medicine, science, and culture*, Cambridge 1993

Cameron, Euan, *Enchanted Europe: superstition, reason, and religion, 1250–1750*, Oxford 2010

Chartier, Roger, *The order of books: readers, authors, and libraries in Europe between the fourteenth and eighteenth centuries*, Cambridge 1994

Christopoulos, John, 'Abortion and the confessional in Counter-Reformation Italy', *RQ* lxv/2 (2012), 443–84

Churchill, Wendy, *Female patients in early modern Britain: gender, diagnosis and treatment*, Farnham 2012

Clark, Stuart, *Thinking with demons: the idea of witchcraft in early modern Europe*, Oxford 1997

Cobb, Matthew, *The egg and sperm race: the seventeenth century scientists who unravelled the secrets of sex, life and growth*, London 2006

Collins, Derek, *Magic in the ancient Greek world*, Oxford 2008

Corfield, Penelope J., 'From poison peddlers to civic worthies: the reputation of the apothecaries in Georgian England', *SHM* xxii/1 (2009), 1–21

Crawford, Patricia, 'Attitudes to menstruation in seventeenth-century England', *P&P* xci (1981), 47–73

—— 'Sexual knowledge in England, 1500–1750', in Porter and Teich, *Sexual knowledge, sexual science*, 82–106

—— *Blood, bodies and families in early modern England*, Harlow 2004

Cressy, David, *Birth, marriage and death: ritual, religion, and the life-cycle in Tudor and Stuart England*, Oxford 2002

Dabhoiwala, Faramerz, *The origins of sex: a history of the first sexual revolution*, Oxford 2012

Darmon, Pierre, *Trial by impotence: virility and marriage in pre-revolutionary France*, trans. Paul Kegan, London 1985

Davies, Kathleen M., 'Continuity and change in literary advice on marriage', in R. B. Outhwaite (ed.), *Marriage and society: studies in the social history of marriage*, London 1981, 58–80

Davies, Owen, *Witchcraft, magic and culture, 1736–1951*, Manchester–New York 1999

—— *Cunning-folk: popular magic in English history*, London 2003

Davies, S. F., 'The reception of Reginald Scot's *Discovery of witchcraft*: witchcraft, magic, and radical religion', *JHI* lxxiv/3 (2013), 381–401

Denninger, Henri Stearns, 'A history of substances known as aphrodisiacs', *Annales of Medical History* ii/4 (1930), 383–93

Dobranski, Stephen, *Readers and authorship in early modern England*, Cambridge 2005

Eccles, Audrey, *Obstetrics and gynaecology in Tudor and Stuart England*, London–Canberra 1982

Elliott, Brent, 'The world of the Renaissance herbal', *Renaissance Studies* xxv/1 (2011), 24–41

Elmer, Peter, *The healing arts: health, disease and society in Europe, 1500–1800*, Manchester 2004

Eshleman, Michael K., 'Diet during pregnancy in the sixteenth and seventeenth centuries', *Journal of the History of Medicine and Allied Sciences* xxx/1 (1975), 23–39

Estes, Leland L., 'Reginald Scot and his *Discoverie of witchcraft*: religion and science in the opposition to the European witch craze', *Church History* lii/4 (1983), 444–56

Evenden Nagy, Doreen, 'Lay and learned medicine in early modern England', in Peter Elmer and Ole Peter Grell (eds), *Health, disease, and society in Europe, 1500–1800: a source book*, Manchester–New York 2004, 38–44

Faraone, Christopher, *Ancient Greek love magic*, Cambridge, MA 2001

Field, Catherine, '"Many hands hands": writing the self in early modern women's recipe books', in M. M. Dowd and J. A. Eckerle (eds), *Genre and women's life writing in early modern England*, Aldershot 2007, 49–63

Findlen, Paula, 'Empty signs? Reading the book of nature in Renaissance science', *Studies in the History and Philosophy of Science* xxi/3 (1990), 511–18

Finucci, Valeria, '"There's the rub": searching for sexual remedies in the New World', *Journal of Medieval and Early Modern Studies* xxxviii/3 (2008), 523–57

Fissell, Mary, 'Gender and generation: representing reproduction in early modern England', *Gender and History* vii/3 (1995), 433–56
—— 'Readers, texts and contexts: vernacular medical works in early modern England', in Roy Porter (ed.), *The popularization of medicine, 1650–1850*, Abingdon 2001, 72–96
—— *Vernacular bodies: the politics of reproduction in early modern England*, Oxford 2004
—— 'The marketplace of print', in Jenner and Wallis, *Medicine and the market*, 108–32
Fitzharris, Lindsey, 'Magic, mysticism and medicine: the medical career of John Webster', in Georganta, Collignon and Millim, *The apothecary's chest*, 119–28
Fletcher, Anthony, *Gender, sex and subordination*, New Haven–London 1995
—— 'Manhood, the male body, courtship and the household in early modern England', *History* lxxxiv/275 (1999), 419–36
Fox, Adam, *Oral and literate culture in England, 1500–1700*, Oxford 1964
Froide, A. M., 'Hidden women: rediscovering the single woman of early modern England', *LPS* lxviii (2002), 26–41
Fumerton, Patricia, 'Remembering by dismembering: databases, archiving, and the recollection of seventeenth-century broadside ballads', in Patricia Fumerton and Anita Guerrini, *Ballads and broadsides in Britain, 1500–1800*, Farnham 2010, 13–34
Furdell, Elizabeth Lane, *Publishing and medicine in early modern England*, New York 2002
Galley, Chris, 'A never-ending succession of epidemics? Mortality in early-modern York', *SHM* vii/1 (1994), 29–57
—— 'The stillbirth rate in early modern England', *LPS* lxxxi (2008), 75–83
Ganev, Robin, 'Milkmaids, ploughmen, and sex in eighteenth-century Britain', *Journal of the History of Sexuality* xvi/1 (2007), 40–67
Gentilcore, David, *Healers and healing in early modern Europe*, Manchester 1998
Georganta, K., F. Collignon and A.-M. Millim (eds), *The apothecary's chest: magic, art and medication*, Newcastle 2009
Gowing, Laura, *Domestic dangers: women, words, and sex in early modern London*, Oxford 1996
—— 'Secret births and infanticide in seventeenth-century England', *P&P* clvi (1997), 87–115
—— *Common bodies: women, touch, and power in seventeenth century England*, New Haven–London 2003
Green, Monica H., 'Review of John M. Riddle, *Eve's herbs*', *Bulletin of the History of Medicine* lxxiii/2 (1999), 308–11
—— 'Bodies, gender, health, disease: recent work on medieval women's medicine', in *Studies in Medieval and Renaissance History: Sexuality and Culture in Medieval and Renaissance Europe* l (2005) 1–46
Gritt, Andy, 'Mortality crisis and household structure: an analysis of parish registers and Compton census, Broughton, Lancashire, 1667–1676', *LPS* lxxix (2007), 38–65
Hackel, Heidi Brayman, *Reading material in early modern England: print, gender and literacy*, Cambridge 2005
Harkness, Deborah, '*Nosce te ipsum*: curiosity, the humoural body and the culture of therapeutics in late sixteenth- and early seventeenth-century England',

in R. J. W. Evans and Alexander Marr (eds), *Curiosity and wonder from the Renaissance to the Enlightenment*, Aldershot 2006, 171–92

Harley, David, 'Spiritual physic, providence and English medicine, 1560–1640', in Ole Peter Grell and Andrew Cunningham (eds), *Medicine and the Reformation*, London–New York 1993, 101–17

Harvey, Karen, *Reading sex in the eighteenth century: bodies and gender in English erotic culture*, Cambridge 2004

Heyd, Uriel, *Reading newspapers: press and public in eighteenth-century Britain and America*, Oxford 2012

Hill Curth, Louise, 'The commercialisation of medicine in the popular press: English almanacs, 1640–1700', *Seventeenth Century* xvii (2002), 48–69

—— 'Medical advertising in the popular press: almanacs and the growth of proprietary medicines', in Hill Curth, *From physick to pharmacology*, 29–47

—— (ed.), *From physick to pharmacology: five hundred years of British drug retailing*, Aldershot 2006

Hindson, Bethan, 'Attitudes towards menstruation and menstrual blood in Elizabethan England', *JSH* xliii/1 (2009), 89–114

Hitchcock, Tim, *English sexualities, 1700–1800*, Basingstoke–London 1997

—— 'The reformulation of sexual knowledge in eighteenth-century England', *Signs* xxvii/4 (2012), 823–31

Hobby, Elaine, *The virtue of necessity: English women's writing, 1649–1688*, London 1988

—— *The birth of mankind: otherwise named, The woman's book*, Farnham 2009

Hufton, Olwen, *The prospect before her: a history of women in Western Europe*, I: *1500–1800*, New York 1995

Hunter, Lynette, 'Women and domestic medicine: lady experimenters, 1570–1620', in Lynette Hunter and Sarah Hutton (eds), *Women, science and medicine, 1500–1700*, Stroud 1997, 89–107

Hunter, Michael, and Annabel Gregory (eds), *An astrological diary of the seventeenth century: Samuel Jeake of Rye, 1652–1699*, Oxford 1988

Ingram, Martin, *Church courts, sex and marriage in England, 1570–1640*, Cambridge 1987

Jacquart, Danielle, and Claude Thomasset, *Sexuality and medicine in the Middle Ages*, trans. Matthew Adamson, Cambridge 1988

Jenner, Mark S. R., and Patrick Wallis, 'The medical market place', in Jenner and Wallis *Medicine and the market*, 1–23

—— (eds), *Medicine and the market in England and its colonies, c. 1450– 1850*, Basingstoke 2007

Johnson, James T., 'English Puritan thought on the ends of marriage', *Church History* xxxviii/4 (1969), 429–36

Jones, R. E., 'Further evidence on the decline in infant mortality in pre-industrial England: North Shropshire, 1561– 1810', *Population Studies* xxxiv/2 (1980), 239–50

Karant-Nunn, Susan C. and Merry E. Wiesner-Hanks (eds), *Luther on women: a sourcebook*, Cambridge 2003

Kieckhefer, Richard, 'Necromancy', in William W. Kibler and Grover A. Zinn (eds), *Medieval France: an encyclopaedia*, New York–London 1995, 661–2

—— *Magic in the Middle Ages*, Cambridge 2000

King, Helen, *The disease of virgins: greensickness, chlorosis and the problems of puberty*, London 2004
Knight, Leah, *Of books and botany in early modern England: sixteenth-century plants and print culture*, Farnham 2009
Kocher, Paul H., *Science and religion in Elizabethan England*, San Marino 1953
Kusukawa, Sachiko, *Picturing the book of nature: image, text, and argument in sixteenth-century human anatomy and medical botany*, Chicago 2012
Laqueur, Thomas, 'Orgasm, generation, and the politics of reproductive biology', *Representations: The Making of the Modern Body: Sexuality and Society in the Nineteenth Century* xiv (1986), 1–41
—— *Making sex: body and gender from the Greeks to Freud*, Cambridge, MA–London 1990
—— 'The rise of sex in the eighteenth century: historical context and historiographical implications', *Signs* xxxvii/4 (2012), 802–12
Laroche, Rebecca, *Medical authority and Englishwomen's herbal texts, 1550–1650*, Farnham 2009
Leong, Elaine, 'Making medicines in the early modern household', *Bulletin of the History of Medicine* lxxxii/1 (2008), 145–68
—— 'Collecting knowledge for the family: recipes, gender and practical knowledge in the early modern English household', *Centaurus* lv/2 (2013), 81–103
—— and Sara Pennell, 'Recipe collections and the currency of medical knowledge in the early modern "marketplace"', in Jenner and Wallis, *Medicine and the market*, 133–52
Lindemann, Mary, *Medicine and society in early modern Europe*, Cambridge 2010
Lindley, David, *The trials of Frances Howard: fact and fiction and the court of King James*, London–New York 1993
McCarl, Mary Rhinelander, 'Publishing the works of Nicholas Culpeper, astrological herbalist and translator of Latin medical works in seventeenth-century London', *Canadian Bulletin of Medical History* xiii/2 (1996), 225–76
McClive, Cathy, 'The hidden truths of the belly: the uncertainties of pregnancy in early modern Europe', *SHM* xv/2 (2002), 209–27
—— 'Menstrual knowledge and medical practice in early modern France, c. 1555–1761', in Shail and Howie, *Menstruation*, 76–89
McConchie, R. W., *Lexicography and physick: the record of sixteenth-century English medical terminology*, Oxford 1997
Macfarlane, Alan, *Marriage and love in England: modes of reproduction, 1300–1840*, Oxford 1986
—— *Witchcraft in Tudor and Stuart England: a regional and comparative study*, London 1999
McLaren, Angus, 'Barrenness against nature: recourse to abortion in pre-industrial England', *Journal of Sex Research* xvii/3 (1981), 224–37
—— *Reproductive rituals: the perception of fertility in England from the sixteenth century to the nineteenth century*, London 1984
—— *Impotence: a cultural history*, Chicago–London 2007
McLaren, Dorothy, 'Fertility, infant mortality, and breastfeeding in the seventeenth century', *Medical History* xxii/4 (1978), 378–96
—— 'Nature's contraceptive: wet-nursing and prolonged lactation: the cases of Chesham, Buckinghamshire, 1578–1601', *Medical History* xxiii/4 (1979), 426–41

Mendleson, Sara, and Patricia Crawford, *Women in early modern England, 1550–1720*, Oxford 1998
Mortimer, Ian, 'The triumph of the doctor: medical assistance to the dying, c. 1570–1720', *Transactions of the Royal Historical Society* xv (2005), 97–116
—— 'The rural medical marketplace in southern England c. 1570–1720', in Jenner and Wallis, *Medicine and the market*, 69–87
Moulton, Ian Frederick, *Before pornography: erotic writing in early modern England*, Oxford 2000
Muir, Edward, *Ritual in early modern Europe*, Cambridge 2005
Nutton, Vivian, '"Prisci dissectionum professores": Greek texts and Renaissance anatomists', in A. C. Dionisotti, Anthony Grafton and Jill Kraye (eds), *The uses of Greek and Latin: historical essays*, London 1988, 111–26
O'Dowd, Michael J., *The history of medications for women: materia medica woman*, New York–London 2001
Peakman, Julie, *Mighty lewd books: the development of pornography in eighteenth-century England*, Basingstoke 2003
Pelling, Margaret, 'Medical practice in early modern England: trade or profession?', in Wilfrid Prest (ed.), *The professions in early modern England*, London 1987, 90–128
—— *Medical conflicts in early modern London: patronage, physicians and irregular practitioners, 1550–1640*, Oxford 2003
Pennell, Sara, 'Perfecting practice? Women, manuscript recipes and knowledge in early modern England', in Victoria E. Burke and Jonathan Gibson (eds), *Early modern women's manuscript writing*, Aldershot 2004, 237–58
Petry, Yvonne, 'Many things surpass our knowledge: an early modern surgeon on magic, witchcraft and demonic possession', *SHM* xxv/1 (2012), 47–64
Porter, Roy, *Health for sale: quackery in England, 1660–1850*, Manchester 1989
—— 'The literature of sexual advice before 1800', in Porter and Teich, *Sexual knowledge, sexual science*, 134–57
—— and Lesley Hall, *The facts of life: the creation of sexual knowledge in Britain, 1650–1950*, New Haven–London 1995
—— and Mikuláš Teich (eds), *Sexual knowledge, sexual science: the history of attitudes to sexuality*, Cambridge–New York 1994
Pullar, Philippa, *Consuming passions: a history of English food and appetites*, London 1970
Raven, James, *The business of books: booksellers and the English book trade, 1450–1850*, New Haven–London 2007
Razzell, Peter, and Christine Spence, 'The history of infant, child and adult mortality in London, 1550–1850', *London Journal* xxxii/3 (2007), 271–92
Read, Sara, *Menstruation and the female body in early modern England*, Basingstoke 2013
Reynolds, L. D., and N. G. Wilson, *Scribes and scholars: a guide to the transmission of Greek and Latin literature*, Oxford 1974
Riddle, John M., 'Oral contraceptives and early-term abortifacients during classical antiquity and the Middle Ages', *P&P* cxxxii (1991), 3–32
—— *Contraception and abortion from the ancient world to the Renaissance*, Cambridge, MA–London 1992
—— *Eve's herbs: a history of contraception and abortion in the West*, Cambridge, MA–London 1997

Rider, Catherine, *Magic and impotence in the Middle Ages*, Oxford 2006
Rosen, Barbara (ed.), *Witchcraft in England, 1558–1618*, Amherst 1991
Rublack, Ulinka, 'Pregnancy, childbirth and the female body in early modern Germany', *P&P* cl/1 (1996), 84–110
Sawday, Jonathan, *The body emblazoned: dissection and the human body in Renaissance culture*, New York–London 1995
Sawyer, Ronald, '"Strangely handled in all her lyms": witchcraft and healing in Jacobean England', *JSH* xxii/3 (1989), 461–85
Schleiner, Winfried, 'Early modern controversies about the one-sex model', *RQ* liii (2000), 180–91
Seaver, Paul S., *Wallington's world: a Puritan artisan in seventeenth-century London*, Stanford 1985
Seeman, Erik R., '"It is better to marry than to burn": Anglo-American attitudes toward celibacy, 1600–1800', *JFH* xxiv/4 (1999), 397–419
Shail, Andrew, and Gillian Howie (eds), *Menstruation: a cultural history*, Basingstoke 2005
Sharpe, James, *Instruments of darkness: witchcraft in England, 1550–1750*, London 1996
Shorter, Edward, *A history of women's bodies*, Harmondsworth 1982
Siena, Kevin P., 'The "foul disease" and privacy: the effects of venereal disease and patient demand on the medical marketplace in early modern London', *Bulletin of the History of Medicine* lxxv/2 (2001), 199–224
Sim, Alison, *Food and feast in Tudor England*, Stroud 2005
Smith, Lisa, 'The relative duties of a man: domestic medicine in England and France, ca. 1685–1740', *JFH* xxxi/3 (2006), 237–56
Solomon, Michael, *Fictions of well-being: sickly readers and vernacular medical writing in late medieval and early modern Spain*, Philadelphia–Oxford 2010
Spufford, Margaret, 'First steps in literacy: the reading and writing experiences of the humblest seventeenth-century spiritual autobiographers', *Social History* iv/3 (1979), 407–35
—— *Small books and pleasant histories; popular fiction and its readership in seventeenth-century England*, Cambridge 1981
Stephens, Walter, 'Witches who steal penises: impotence and illusion in *Malleus maleficarum*', *Journal of Medieval and Early Modern Studies* xxviii/3 (1998) 495–516
—— *Demon lovers: witchcraft, sex and the crisis of belief*, Chicago–London 2002
Stolberg, Michael, 'A woman down to her bones: the anatomy of sexual difference in the sixteenth and early seventeenth centuries', *Isis* xcii (2003), 274–99
—— 'Menstruation and sexual difference in early modern medicine', in Shail and Howie, *Menstruation*, 90–101
Stone, Lawrence, *The family, sex and marriage in England, 1500–1800*, London 1990
Taavitsainen, Irma, Peter Murray Jones, Paivi Pahta, Turo Hiltunen, Ville Marttila, Maura Rtia, Carla Suhr and Jukka Tyrkko, 'Medical texts in 1500–1700 and the corpus of early modern English medical texts', in Irma Taavitsainen and Paivi Pahta (eds), *Medical writing in early modern English*, Cambridge 2011, 9–25

Tague, Ingrid, 'Aristocratic women and ideas of family in the early eighteenth century', in Berry and Foyester, *The family in early modern England*, 184–208
Thirsk, Joan, *Food in early modern England*, London 2007
Thomas, Keith, *Religion and the decline of magic*, London 1991
Thompson, Roger, 'Popular reading and humour in Restoration England', *Journal of Popular Culture* ix/3 (1975), 653–71
Thorndike, Lynn, *A History of magic and experimental science*, VI: *The sixteenth century*, New York–London 1966
Totelin, Laurence, 'Sex and vegetables in the Hippocratic gynaecological treatises', *Studies in History and Philosophy of Science, part C: Studies in History and Philosophy of Biological and Biomedical Sciences* xxxviii/3 (2007), 531–40
—— *Hippocratic recipes: oral and written transmission of pharmacological knowledge in fifth and fourth century Greece*, Leiden–Boston 2009
Toulalan, Sarah, *Imagining sex: pornography and bodies in seventeenth-century England*, Oxford 2007
—— 'To[o] much eating stifles the child: fat bodies and reproduction in early modern England, *Historical Research* lxxxvii (2014), 65–93
—— '"Unfit for generation": body size and reproduction', in Raymond Stephanson and Darren Wagner (eds), *The secrets of generation: reproduction in the long eighteenth century*, Toronto 2014
Traister, Barbara, '"Matrix and the pain thereof": a sixteenth-century gynaecological essay', *Medical History* xxxv/4 (1991), 436–51
van de Walle, Etienne, 'Flowers and fruits: two thousand years of menstrual regulation', *Journal of Interdisciplinary History* xxviii/2 (1997), 183–203
—— and Elisha P. Renne (eds), *Regulating menstruation: beliefs, practices, interpretations*, Chicago 2001
Van Ruler, J. A., 'Minds, forms, and spirits: the nature of Cartesian disenchantment', *JHI* lxi/3 (2000), 381–95
Vann, Richard T., 'Unnatural infertility, or, whatever happened in Colyton? Some reflections on *English population history from family reconstitution, 1580–1837*', *Continuity and Change* xiv/1 (1999), 91–104
Viazzo, Pier Paolo, 'Mortality, fertility, and family', trans. Caroline Beamish, in David I. Kertzer and Marzio Barbagli (eds), *The history of the European family*, I: *Family life in early modern times, 1500–1789*, New Haven–London 2001, 157–87
Wallis, Patrick, 'Apothecaries and the consumption and retailing of medicines in early modern London', in Hill Curth, *From physick to pharmacology*, 13–27
—— 'Exotic drugs and English medicine: England's drug trade, c. 1550–c. 1800' *SHM* xxv/1 (2012), 20–46
Walton, Alan Hull, *Aphrodisiacs from legend to prescription: a study of aphrodisiacs throughout the ages, with sections on suitable food, glandular extracts, hormone stimulation and rejuvenation*, Westport, CN 1958
Watt, Tessa, *Cheap print and popular piety, 1550–1640*, Cambridge 1991
Wear, Andrew, *Knowledge and practice in English medicine, 1550–1680*, Cambridge 2000
Webster, Charles, 'Paracelsus confronts the saints: miracles, healing and the secularization of magic', *SHM* viii/3 (1995), 403–21
Wrigley, E. A., 'Explaining the rise in marital fertility in England in the "long" eighteenth century', *Economic History Review* li/3 (1998), 435–64

Unpublished dissertations

Evans, Jennifer 'Procreation, pleasure and provokers of lust in early modern England, 1550–1780', PhD Exeter 2010

Oren-Magidor, Daphna, '"Make me a fruitfull vine": dealing with infertility in early modern England', PhD Brown 2012

Index

Abbott, George, 152, 156
abortion, 42, 161–5, 171–4, 177–8; abortifacients, 10, 173; as contraception, 161–2; to prevent, 42, 180, 184; as a term for miscarriage, 175–6; women's knowledge of, 162
adultery, 1, 19, 22, 129. *See also* cuckolds.
advertisements, 2, 32, 47–9, 96–8, 102, 193
anatomical discoveries, 60–1; influence on theories of infertility, 77, 107
animalcules, 60–1, 77, 107
aphrodisiacs: birds, 91, 101, 102–4, 113–14, 117, 119, 120, 121, 179–80; flatulent, 11, 104, 109–16; heating, 90–100, 103, 113, 129, 154, 166, 168, 172, 180–4, 188, 194; language used of, 3–6; nourishing, 41, 100–8, 109, 112, 113, 120, 129, 177, 180–4; salty, 93, 105–7; seed-producing, 102–5; signature, 11, 12, 103, 116–27, 154; ungendered nature of, 88–9, 91, 97–8, 111–13, 117–18, 119, 128; use in emmenagogues, 173–4; as witchcraft treatment, 151–6
apothecary, 9, 12, 32, 38, 45, 47, 137, 161, 169
Aristotle's/Aristoteles master-piece, 37, 41, 51, 127, 179
Astruc, Jean, 4, 74, 87

ballads, 1, 2, 22–3, 42–4
barrenness, *see* infertility
Barrough, Philip, 65
Bonet, Theophile, 4, 65
Braganza, Catherine of (wife of Charles II, king of Great Britain), 7, 20, 24–5
breastfeeding, 14–15
Burnet, Gilbert, 20

camphor, 81, 156, 192
cantharides, 10, 47, 96, 98–9, 127, 155, 169
Cartesian rationalism, 145–6
caudle, 1, 113–14, 119, 120

child mortality rates, 15–16, 193
conception: agricultural metaphors, 40, 64, 129–30; gender roles in, 59–61, 165; impediments to, *see* fertility; indicators of, 78; knowledge of, 40–1, 46; simultaneous orgasm, 59–60, 78. *See also* infertility; seed.
Crooke, Helkiah, 53
cuckolds, 21–2, 43, 136
Culpeper, Nicholas, 32–3, 34, 35, 65, 181

demography, 13–18, 24–5
Devereux, Robert, 3rd earl of Essex, 156–7
divorce, 20, 75. *See also* impotence.
domestic medicine, 45–6, 118–19, 169
Drage, William, 38, 137, 142

erectile dysfunction, *see* impotence
erotic literature, 40–2
Essex, Robert Devereux, 3rd earl of, *see* Devereux, Robert

fertility, 92–3, 163, 164, 170, 193; beyond conception, 27, 160, 175, 177, 180, 185, 187, 188, 189; excessive, 62; importance in marriage, 21, 23–4; patent remedies for, 96–8; regulated by God, 24, 61–2, 67–8, 131, 144, 152; rural fecundity, 25. *See also* aphrodisiacs; demography; infertility; menstruation and fertility; seed.
Flower family, 132, 157–8
Freke, Elizabeth, 45
frigidity, 21, 72–4, 87, 90, 194

Gerard, John, 38, 94, 95, 185
Germane, Maria, 53
Gouge, William, 19

health: regulated by God, 68, 157–8, 187
heat: as a cause of infertility, 68–9; as a determinant of gender, 52–3, 99–100. *See also* aphrodisiacs, heating.
herbals, 14, 34, 37–8, 94, 95, 184, 185–6

213

Howard, Frances, 131, 152, 156–7, 158
humours: humoural body, 5, 46, 51–2, 64, 98, 110, 159; humoural framework, 2, 13, 16, 74, 88; humoural imbalance, 7, 68–71, 76–8, 83, 166, 177–8, 181; humoural virtues of plants, 94, 161, 171–2, 181

impotence: erectile dysfunction, 65, 82, 84, 85–6; as grounds for annulment, 21, 75; and infertility, 44, 49, 80, 85–6, 128; and masculinity, 22–3; terminology, 63–6, 76, 78, 97–8. See also witchcraft.
infertility: biblical discussions of, 6, 21, 64, 68, 191; and body weight, 71, 82, 112; causes, 25, 26, 51, 67–86, 133–5, 137–9, 192–3; effects on social roles, 23–4, 44; gendered terminology, 26, 63–6, 191; legal discussions of, 20–1; tests, 42; treatments for, 6–8, 26, 48, 87–129, 147–56, 174. See also witchcraft.

Laqueur, Thomas, 52, 55, 74, 128, 191, 193
Lemnius, Laevinus, 19, 37, 114
love, 20, 73
lust, 6, 18–19, 24, 89–90, 195; as a cause of miscarriage, 177, 180, 188; regulation of, 81, 156–57. See also sexual pleasure.
luxury, 17, 25

McLaren, Angus, 11–12, 23–4, 27, 133, 161, 162, 163, 178
magic, see witchcraft.
Manners, Francis, 6th earl of Rutland, 157–8
manuscript recipe collections, 26, 34, 38–40, 91, 94–5, 169, 171, 181
marriage, 18–24, 43, 140, 191, 194; age at time of, 13, 58; consummation, 156
Marten, John, 4, 104
masculinity, see impotence
Massaria, Alessandro, 103
medical marketplace, 26, 44–50, 191–2; access to physicians, 46
medical texts: book trade, 30–3, 37, 50; evolution of ideas in, 36–7, 77–8, 85, 115, 191; readership, 32, 33–6
medicines: as specifics, 87, 180, 184
menstruation: emmenagogues, 27, 161, 173–4, as fertility remedies, 168–71, humoural virtues of, 171–3, interpretations of, 161–5; and fertility, 165–8; lack of, 71–2, 165; menarche, 93, 160; menstrual blood, 57–8, 62–3, 165; menstrual regularity, 164, 166–7, 168; and sexual pleasure, 167–8. See also abortion, abortifacients.
miscarriage, 14, 27, 160, 175–88, 193; terminology, 175–6
More, Thomas, 155

one-sex model, 52–6, 64, 88, 110, 128. See also Laqueur, Thomas.

Paracelsian medicine, 32, 116, 132, 138, 181
Paré, Ambrose, 8, 104
Pechey, John, 186
Perkins, William, 19
population, see demography
pornography, see erotic literature
prayer: as a treatment for infertility, 68, 132, 147, 148, 149, 151–2, 192
premature ejaculation, 11, 66, 80–1
privacy, see secrecy
prostitutes, 1, 2, 40, 41, 102, 120, 125
Protestantism: views on illness, 67–8, 132; views on sexuality, 19

Raynalde, Thomas, 37, 67, 69
Riverius, Lazarus, 34
Ross, Alexander, 55
Royal College of Physicians, 4, 31, 32, 38, 185, 186
rural sexuality, 25
Rutland, Francis Manners, 6th earl of, see Manners, Francis

Sadler, John, 59, 177
Scot, Reginald, 144, 148, 149
secrecy, 49, 169, 193
seed, 56–9; and bodyweight, 71; discovery of spermatozoa and eggs, 60–1, 77; flatulent nature of, 109; gendered nature of, 36, 57–9, 62–3; incompatibility of, 75; salty nature of, 56–7, 79, 93, 105–7; stimulating qualities of, 51, 59, 78–81, 92, 104–5, 108; weakness of 66, 74–8, 84, 114
sex: illicit 17, 129, 194; sexual liberalism, 6, 128–9, 193–4
sexual pleasure, 6, 11, 18–20, 25, 26,

43, 56, 74, 78, 86, 87, 89–90, 128, 129, 194; and conception, 59, 78, 128–9, 193; God as creator of, 19, 89, 129; and heat, 74, 90, 92, 95–6; lack of, 67, 73–4, 79, 81, 143. *See also* aphrodisiacs; frigidity; menstruation; seed, stimulating nature of.
Sharp, Jane, 37, 55, 65, 179
single women, 162–3
Spanish Fly, *see* cantharides

Thomas, Keith, 132, 151, 159
two-sex model, 52, 55–6, 88, 98, 128
  See also Laqueur, Thomas.

upper classes, 7, 16, 24–5, 158

venereal disease, 5, 49
virago, 53, 71, 92
vital spirits, 11, 16, 74, 75, 77, 82, 86, 97, 134

Wallington, Nehemiah, 1–2
wind: as a cause of erection, 85, 115; in the womb, 110, 112, 178, 182–3
windy foods, *see* aphrodisiacs, flatulent
witchcraft, 27, 131–59; boundaries with natural magic, 132, 135–7; cunning-folk, 132, 138, 148, 151, 159, 192; enchantment, 133, 138, 140, 141–3, 147, 157–8; familiars, 142, 157; ligature spell, 139–41; medieval precedents, 133–4, 152–3; permanence of spells, 158; ritualistic responses to, 133, 148–51, 153; scepticism of, 144–7, 151–2
womb, 61–2; active nature of, 61, 74; anatomical diagrams of, 52–3; humoural condition of, 68–70; physical deformities, 70–1; structure 61

www.ingramcontent.com/pod-product-compliance
Lightning Source LLC
Chambersburg PA
CBHW070803230426
43665CB00017B/2471